Ivar Johansen

S0-BNZ-309

PNI

PNI

THE NEW
MIND / BODY
HEALING PROGRAM

Elliott S. Dacher, M.D.

PARAGON HOUSE
90 Fifth Avenue, New York, NY 10011

First paperback edition, 1993

Published in the United States by

Paragon House
90 Fifth Avenue
New York, N. Y. 10011

Copyright © 1991 by Elliott Dacher

All rights reserved. No part of this book may be
reproduced, in any form, without written permission from
the publishers, unless by a reviewer who wishes
to quote brief passages.

Library of Congress Cataloging-in-Publishing data

Dacher, Elliott S.,
PNI : the new mind-body healing program / Elliott S. Dacher. —
1st ed.
p.   cm.
Includes bibliographical references and index.
ISBN 1-55778-468-X (HC)
ISBN 1-55778-599-6 (Pbk)
1. Mind and body.   2. Health.   3. Psychoneuroimmunology.
I. Title.
RA776.5.D324   1991
613—dc20   91-11563
CIP

10   9   8   7   6   5   4   3   2

For
DORA AND HARRY
Whose sacrifices gave birth to my life
and
JESSICA AND ALISON
Whose lives give meaning to mine

CONTENTS

INTRODUCTION   xiii

1. THE LIMITS OF MODERN MEDICINE:
   FRONTIERS OF HEALING   1

2. PSYCHONEUROIMMUNOLOGY:
   RECONNECTING MIND AND BODY   15

3. MINDFULNESS   30

4. SELF-REGULATION   57

5. ACHIEVING GENERAL RELAXATION   69

6. REGULATING THE BODY   85

7. REGULATING THE MIND   118

8. WORKING THE PROGRAM   153

9. NAVIGATING THE HEALTH-CARE SYSTEM   171

10. THE FOUR STAGES OF HEALING   189

    NOTES   197

    BIBLIOGRAPHY   201

    RESOURCES   209

    INDEX   211

ACKNOWLEDGMENTS

Projects such as this are never done alone. Many thanks are due. Dr. Jean Houston first showed me what was possible, and Dr. Rudolph Bauer held the light at the darkest hours. Krishnamurti taught me about the pathless path, and Patanjali provided it. Many assisted in the practical details. Anita DeVivo's help in editing and structuring the initial manuscript was invaluable. My agent John White's faith in the book inspired me to continue, and Andy DeSalvo at Paragon House read it, understood it, and brought it to print. Finally, among the many who offered constant encouragement and goodwill are Milton Friedman, Peggy Heller, Brenda Sanchez, Kay Stoller, Neal Vahle, Riva Wine, Metadocs, and those whose unconditional love breached the walls and opened my heart.

EXERCISES

INTRODUCTION TO THE EXERCISES   40

1. MIND-TALK   41

2. MINDFULNESS   45

3. TRAINING YOURSELF IN MINDFULNESS   51

4. A MODIFIED MINDFULNESS TRAINING EXERCISE
(FOR INDIVIDUALS WITH A RESTLESS MIND)   53

5. MINDFULNESS (IN DAILY LIVING)   54

6. TENSE-RELAX   75

7. CONTROLLED BREATHING (1)   77

8. GUIDED IMAGERY   81

9. THE RESPIRATORY SYSTEM   90

10. CONTROLLED BREATHING (2)   92

11. THE CARDIOVASCULAR SYSTEM   99

12. THE GASTROINTESTINAL SYSTEM   106

13. THE IMMUNE SYSTEM   112

14. DISCOVERING INNER POWER   128

15. GRIEVING OUR LOSSES   131

16. MINDFUL RELATIONSHIPS   141

17. OBSERVING DEPRIVATION AND ABUNDANCE   148

18. REMEMBERING   149

INTRODUCTION

I WAS EIGHT years old when I first knew I wanted to be a doctor. Perhaps this desire grew out of my childhood experience with the doctor who came to the house when I was ill. He was patient and had time to talk while waiting to sterilize a needle in boiling water on our kitchen stove. He brought a sense of comfort and caring, wisdom and authority, softness and sensitivity. It seemed to me that he knew something about my life, and I felt secure in his presence. He knew my family well, and that, too, seemed important.

Fourteen years later I entered medical school and began the first phase of becoming a healer: assimilating the knowledge and learning the techniques of the physician-scientist. Bursting with enthusiasm, I welcomed this opportunity. My fellow students and I learned about anatomy and physiology, pharmacology and biochemistry, physical diagnosis and treatment. Finally, after the first two years were over, we were on the hospital wards with real patients. Shortly after, we scattered around the country for internships, residencies, and, eventually, the practice of medicine.

"Eventually" came sooner than I thought. Working as an internist in a Health Maintenance Organization (HMO), I discovered I was expected to see twenty-five to thirty patients each day, complete paper work, answer and return phone calls, and attend meetings. This left an average of six to ten minutes for each patient. At the end of the first year I was frustrated and disillusioned with how mechanical and automatic practicing medicine had become; I was placing Band-Aids on problems rather than resolving them.

Thus began the second phase of my becoming a healer. As I began to read about prevention, stress, wellness, and holism a new world opened for me. I traveled around the country to meet the leaders in these fields and introduced this new information into my practice and, to a lesser degree, I was to learn later, into my life. I slowly became a local expert on these subjects and was appointed director of the health promotion program at the HMO. I thought I finally understood the nature of health and healing. It is always at times of such arrogance that one courts the great fall.

In a very short span of time, several critical events occurred in my life. First, in learning about the healing practices of the ancient Greek Aesclepian healing temples, I discovered a way to approach healing that was richer and deeper than the medical training I already knew. Then, in a close personal relationship I experienced, for the first time, the grace and mystery of unconditional love. My heart opened in a way I had long forgotten. I began to feel my life rather than think it, finally acknowledging my unhappiness and disillusionment with all that had come before. For me, these events closed a phase of my life and began the third and critical phase of my becoming a healer.

At that point, a "huge dark hole" opened in my existence and nothing that I had previously known as my life seemed to work. I began to hear the long-denied voice of my youth, which still remembered the feeling of joy and delight unencumbered by fear and defensiveness. Within a few months, my life was in turmoil. My long-term job, relationship, and personality (as I had known it) were gone. I entered a period of chaos, disorientation, and pain that was beyond anything that can be expressed in words and is known only to those who enter such emptiness.

It took more than a year to heal myself. During this period, when the last remnants of my previous life were gone, I experienced a sort of death, and, in a strange and mysterious way, in this death, in this abysmal nothingness, I met myself in a very different way. This self had no form, no name, no concept, no life, no death, nothing—just a sense of presence and being.

Slowly and painfully, with reading, studying, meditation, and guidance, I began to know a deeper part of myself, and tentatively returned to life. During this process I was to learn the more profound aspects of the art of the healer. I learned about compassion through the painful recognition that what separates my situation in life from that of any other person is no more than the time between two heartbeats. I learned about self-responsibility when I saw my own dying, and knew that, after my friends did all they could, only I could choose life, get up, and start learning to walk again. When I did, I began to learn about living in the present moment, which suddenly becomes easy when there appears to be no past or future available.

I learned about how to live with emotions rather than run from them. I learned about my mind and its illusions and distortions. I learned about faith, spirit, and, most important, about love, without which there is no healing. I learned how to be a very different healer, and returned to a new and sacred vision of healing.

I entered the fourth phase of becoming a healer when I resumed my role as a physician. A strange thing happened as I returned to this calling. I was able to accept medicine just as I had learned it in medical school. This was possible because I now knew scientific medicine often needed to be a part of healing, and I no longer demanded more of it than it could deliver. I began to bring into my practice all of the aspects of healing that I had learned in my training—*all* of my training.

My relationships with patients changed. We began a journey to health rather than a problem-oriented medical encounter. Each journey was different. I explored the mixture of scientific medicine, meditation, imagery, biofeedback, nutrition, and that special kind of love and commitment shared by those assisting each other in healing. Some years later I learned about the research in a new field of medical inquiry: psychoneuroimmunology (PNI). This was an exciting discovery of the unfolding scientific validation of the mind-body work I practice daily in my office.

Slowly, a new kind of medicine is emerging. This medicine of the future is already here in its early form. It is challenging us to move beyond our limits and to use our extraordinary human capacities for self-directed healing: capacities we now know are under our conscious control.

I have written this book to share with you the ideas and practices of this "new medicine." Together we will explore and learn about the emerging field of PNI and the research that is demonstrating and documenting the amazing capacity of *each of our minds* to self-regulate and self-direct our lives. We will discover how it is possible for all individuals to prevent, reverse, and heal disease by undertaking a program of self-healing. More importantly, we will learn how to expand our lives and achieve full health; not merely the absence of disease but the vitality and aliveness that for too many of us is an occasional "accident" rather than a way of life.

This book is designed as a workbook and training program, an ongoing course in healing. It is designed to assist you in inquiring into your life and discovering your unique and untapped capacities for full health. It provides you with essential state-of-the-art information and exercises that I use every day in my workshops and practice. The exercises have enabled individuals such as you to expand upon the text by directly experiencing and verifying each of its ideas and approaches.

We begin by exploring the important differences between treatment, the use of outside resources to reduce or eliminate the signs and symptoms of illness, and healing, the use of your natural inner capacities to achieve full health. You will then be introduced to and taught the two components of healing; mindfulness and self-regulation. You will learn how mindfulness, a powerful, yet largely unknown, capacity of the mind that is available to each individual, can provide us with insight, creativity, and extraordinary healing powers. Using mindfulness, you will discover that it is possible to self-regulate and heal the mind and body in a manner that, although known for millenia by healers and mystics, is for the first time being rediscovered by scientists and made available to those who seek it. The final part of the book will assist you in integrating these capacities into your daily life, and creating a program for long-term growth and health.

Professionals and professionals-in-training do not have the luxury of continuing education and training curriculums that teach the principles of mind-body healing. Dazzled by the wonders of modern technology, our mentors have lost sight of the special technology that is built in to each of us. It is for us to teach ourselves and then teach our teachers. This book can serve as an introduction and guide to the new medicine that your clients will increasingly demand, and as an opportunity to create a personal and professional life that lives the healing we desire to teach.

Read a chapter, practice an exercise, and linger with what you discover. Carefully begin to observe your life and determine how this information fits into your daily activities. As you will notice, the simplest act—tying your shoe laces, brushing your teeth—is an opportunity to fine-tune and train your mind. This is not a book to read and put down. It is not an end in itself. It must come alive in your life as you discover and experiment with your natural healing capacity. Slowly you will come to honor the brilliance of your mind and body as your foremost authority and resource. If you are ready to heal your life, slowly you will write your own book and orchestrate your own healthy future.

As I work with this information in my own life, one-to-one in my practice, and in workshops, I have come to know the power that is available to each of us when we learn and use these simple, yet profound, natural capacities. This is not the power to control and manipulate other people or things but the power to tap into the most profound wisdom of the ages, to become a midwife to one's own rebirthing and cocreator of all that is best in human life. As we go down this path together, I imagine that you and I will begin to touch into the deeper mysteries of life and the elusive, but most important of human opportunities: love, joy, peace, and freedom.

Fall, 1990
Martha's Vineyard

Chapter 1

THE LIMITS OF
MODERN MEDICINE:
FRONTIERS OF HEALING

ON THE SURFACE, some moments in life appear uneventful. When revisited, from the perspective of intervening years, they assume a meaning of great importance. Such a moment, etched as an image on my mind, occurred the afternoon of my first day in medical school.

On that particular day, the entering students, all one hundred of us, were taken as a group to the local Veterans Administration hospital. We marched proudly into the auditorium, sat down in hushed anticipation, and the dean of students said, "We are going to bring in your first patient." An elderly man in a bathrobe was led to the center of the stage. Addressing us, the dean said, "Tell me what disease this man has."

There was a second of silence, and then our questions started popping. We wanted to know if the man had a pain here, a pain there. The man answered all kinds of questions as best he could. He was direct and succinct; he must have had some experience with such demonstrations.

1

After fifteen minutes one of the students made the diagnosis: "He has an ulcer."

The dean nodded with pride. "Yes, he does. . . . That is wonderful! See how good you already are as physicians, and you have not even gone through medical school."

So here was the first lesson I learned as a doctor-to-be: ask for symptoms, make a diagnosis, and treat the symptoms. From those first moments in medical school I learned to focus on disease rather than health, pathology rather than the person, parts rather than the whole, an ulcer rather than an ulcerated life.

During the next four years, we learned to perfect our skills in this area: to take a medical history, perform examinations, differentiate among a constellation of symptoms, and, of course, treat the disease or ailment. When we graduated, we were the products of an expensive, thorough, and excellent education in the treatment of disease. We had an ever-expanding technical arsenal and a knowledge of hundreds of drugs to help us treat the sick.

We traveled across the country to internships and residencies. Finally, the day came; our training was complete, and we began to practice medicine. In private practice, at a university, or in a health plan, we were ready for our first patients.

THE PATIENT GETS TRAINED, TOO

As a consumer of medical care, you receive training, too. You have learned that, if you are troubled or ill and in need of diagnosis and treatment, you must first check your health insurance card and then call your health plan or physician's office for an appointment. The physician you call will likely be a primary-care physician or a specialist limiting his or her practice to a specific anatomical area: foot, heart, bone, etc. Your ticket of admission is a symptom, preferably a physical symptom. Those symptoms that receive the most urgent attention involve blood, pain, or a lump. You leave for your appointment with a mixture of apprehension, expectation, and relief. The office, more than likely in a nondescript sterile building furnished with generic tables, chairs, and outdated magazines, is watched over by the office staff, who are well separated from you by an impenetrable glass wall.

When your turn arrives, you enter the doctor's consultation room, nervously find your chair and take note of the diplomas and licensure conspicuously placed on the wall. Each testifies to the training and professional status of the physician, assuring you that the physician is scientifically trained, tested, and certified.

The physician enters. He or she checks your chart, nods in your direction and asks, "What's wrong?" More than likely, you will relate the events leading to your visit with a focus on physical symptoms. Listening to your history, your physician, trained to synthesize these symptoms into categories called symptom complexes, which identify specific diseases, leads you into the examination room to complete a physical examination, which may include blood and urine tests, an electrocardiogram, and, potentially, a variety of other appropriate procedures or tests.

Your symptoms and examination findings may result in an interim diagnosis or a specific therapy. However, further tests or the opinion of another specialist may be required. If all the tests are normal, and your symptoms are nonspecific, you will be reassured, dismissed, and considered one of the "worried well" (a term used by health professionals to describe individuals who feel unhealthy but whose physical examination and laboratory tests are normal).

If therapy is initiated, you will be expected to comply with the recommendations and report back any side effects, as well as the outcome of treatment. If treatment is successful, your symptoms will regress, and you will return to life as usual, interacting with the physician only when another problem emerges to disturb your normal activities or body feelings. For the most part, this is the way healing is done today.

TEMPLE HEALING: A LESSON FROM THE PAST

How far have we come from our ancient healing practices? If you had lived in 500 B.C. and were ill or troubled, physically or emotionally, and in need of healing, you would have journeyed to Cos, Epidaurus, Pergamon, or one of the many other temples of the ancient Greek healing god, Aesclepias. * You would have participated in practices that

---

*I was first introduced to Aesclepian healing by Dr. Jean Houston.

continued without interruption from 500 B.C. to 300 A.D. throughout Europe, the Near East, and the Mediterranean, where temple medicine was the foremost source of healing.

Your decision to journey to the temple would not be made lightly; healing was a sacred process—a communion with self and the gods. After consulting friends and physician, you would prepare to leave for the healing temple. The journey of several days would be interrupted with stories of miracle cures from those returning home. With rising hope and expectation you arrive at the temple gates. Here you would read testimonials etched in stone, such as:

> Believe me, men, I have been dead all the years I have been alive. The beautiful, the good, the holy, the evil were all the same to me; such it seems was the darkness that formerly enveloped my understanding and concealed and hid from me all these things. But now that I have come here, I have become alive, as if I had laid down in the temple of Aesclepias and been saved. I walk, I talk, I think. The sun so great, so beautiful. I have now discovered men, for the first time: now I see the clear sky, you, the air, the acropolis, the theater. [PAPYRUS DIDOTRANA (approximately 360 B.C.)]

> . . . lame. He came as a supplicant, to the sanctuary on a stretcher. In his sleep he saw a vision. It seemed to him that the God broke his crutch and ordered him to get a ladder and climb as high as possible. He dared to carry it out . . . and walked out unhurt. (fourth century B.C.)

Upon your arrival you would begin the process of purification through cleansing and fasting; a symbolic shedding of toxic attitudes and the unhealthy habits of daily life. At this point, you would become part of a dynamic and varied healing environment. Walking in the temple grounds, you would enjoy the beautiful gardens and the graceful and serene statues of the great Greek sculptors Phidias and Praxiteles. Roaming minstrels would lift your spirit, and you would participate in lively philosophical dialogues that would stimulate your intellect and challenge you to consider alternate perspectives to your current life situation.

You might attend dramatic performances such as the tragedies of Aeschylus, Euripides, or Sophocles, which portray the cycles and rhythms of human life and teach that we share life and human nature with our fellow humans, suffering together our pain and distress as part of life's movement toward knowledge, maturity, and healing; or you might have a massage, participate in an athletic competition, or consult the priests regarding diet or the use of herbs or pharmaceuticals of the time.

Each evening, dressed in your ceremonial white robes, you would gather with others in the sacred temple to leave offerings to Aesclepias as you bid him to visit you at night with a healing dream. In the morning, you or some other petitioner may awake healed. Others might relate the content of their dreams to priests who would assist in interpretation and provide instruction in dieting and the use of medicinals.

Day after day, removed from the stress and pulls of daily life, focusing on diet, fitness, relaxation, and self-examination, you would experience a slow return of energy and vitality. Finally, the day would arrive when you felt restored with a sense of wholeness, balance, and harmony, ready for your return home. Immersed in activities for mind, body, and spirit, you would have learned about yourself and developed new attitudes and behaviors—healthy, life-supporting ones.

As illogical as it may seem to our scientific minds, we can accept that many of the visitors to the temples returned home with renewed health. The continued existence of the temples for eight hundred years, the personal testimonials of healings, and the written words of the great philosophers and writers of ancient Greece support this conclusion. Some may have returned to health as a result of the natural history of their disease, others may have improved from the relaxed environment, pharmaceuticals, exercise, nutritional practices, community support, a shift in perspective, and the inevitable healing that comes from the release of the tensions of daily life.

Of greater significance is the fundamental approach of the healing temples, which viewed the individual as a whole person and emphasized the interactive unity of mind and body. Neither mind nor body was treated alone. Both were considered as aspects of the total human organism, the mind-body. This holistic view, an essential aspect of Greek humanism, allowed a natural evolution of holistic healing practices using science, the arts, philosophy, humor, and spirituality to replace stress with harmony, anger with peace, despair with hope, mental paralysis with possibility, and isolation with community.

Lacking a technical knowledge of physical diagnosis and therapy, the

ancient practitioners of medicine were compelled to use their understanding of the human mind and spirit to heal the body. The
individual—his or her attitudes, beliefs, and behavior—were inescap-
ably central to the healing process.

IS ANCIENT HISTORY REVISITING US?

You do not have to go very far from your own home to rediscover in
modern society the essential elements of the Aescelpian healing temples. Every day, in a church, school, or other meeting area in your
community, you can visit an Alcoholics Anonymous (AA) meeting
with the million or so others who do so each day around the world. It is
ironic that, twenty-five hundred years after Aesclepias, alcoholism, a
disease that accounts for a substantial number of hospitalizations and
deaths in twentieth-century America, is best treated through the
twelve-step spiritual cure of AA. Alcoholics and their physicians,
unable to successfully treat or heal this disease with all of the technology of modern medicine, rejoin their Aesclepian ancestors in turning to
a more holistic approach.

The principles of AA, which are now extended to many similar
groups coping with a variety of disorders, emphasize a disciplined and
committed process of recovery through self-directed actions that range
from self-investigation and life-style change to attitudinal healing and
conscious living. The reader may respond by saying, "This is an emotional problem." Ask an alcoholic. It is a mind-body problem.

Another good example of the bridging of mind and body was reported in a 1977 issue of the *Journal of The American Medical Association*
(JAMA).[1] A Philippine-American suffering from a severe case of lupus,
a disease involving many parts of the body, became despondent with the
progression of her illness, which seemed unresponsive to medications.
There could be no question, according to the report, of the severity of
her disease, the involvement of multiple body organs, or the progressive
advancement of her disease even while she was on the most powerful
medications.

She returned to her native village seeking further help with the
disease. Two weeks later, following the removal of a curse by a local
witch doctor, she arrived back in her American physician's office appar-

ently cured. To her physician's amazement she did not even suffer the usual withdrawal symptoms from her powerful medicines. Five years later she remained completely disease free.

Although this case was reported in a major medical journal, it was likely considered by most physicians as an interesting anomaly. This, despite the fact, that many similar reports can be found in the medical literature. It is ironic that we are so absorbed with miracles of another kind, modern technology, that we have lost trust, faith, and knowledge of the extraordinary healing powers of the human mind, body, and spirit. As we have invested in the miracle of technology, we have disinvested in the miracle of our humanness.

In this new age of scientific wonders, technology makes it possible for us to attain precise pictures of the inner workings of the human body, measure infinitesimal metabolic reactions, exchange organs from one person to another, grow babies in test tubes, and maintain physiologic life when all signs of human life are gone. Our approach to health and disease has resulted in diagnostic and therapeutic capacities that are unparalleled in human history. These achievements have enabled us to alter successfully the natural history of many diseases and to provide helpful treatment in others. Nothing can detract from these accomplishments. Yet scientific medicine is at its limits when confronting degenerative and stress-related diseases, which are more related to the way we think and live than to bacteria, viruses, and toxins. These problems of living cannot be analyzed under a microscope, cured with medicines, excised with a scalpel or eliminated through organ transplants. They cannot be reduced to biophysiology or comprehended by separate medical specialities.

Consider John's "medical problem." He is thirty-four years old. He came to my office with the understanding that I work with certain medical problems in a different way. For the past five years, he had been suffering with moderate symptoms from a disease called ulcerative colitis, a chronic, recurrent ulceration of the colon. He had been on a variety of medications, at times responding so that he was free of symptoms for many months at a time. Nevertheless, he continued to suffer with no permanent end to the problem in sight, even though he had received good medical care and was treated with proper medications.

The exacerbations and remissions of his illness were consistent with the medical understanding of this problem and with the acknowledged fact that there was no cure for his disease, only treatment. He had reached the limits of conventional medicine's capacity to improve his disease, and was instructed to use the medicines as needed and live with it as best as possible. That, however, was not good enough for John. He wanted to be healed.

In our meeting, I discussed with John the mind-body approach to illness and the effort it would require of him. I asked him if he would be willing to work with me in looking at his illness from a different perspective; a self-healing perspective that expands upon conventional treatment. He agreed. I explained to him that it would be helpful to use a relaxation technique, which clears the mind and allows access to hidden information stored in the mind, and mental imagery, which often assists in bringing this information to awareness. I instructed and guided John into deep relaxation. When I could observe through his breathing, complexion, and body posture that he had entered a relaxed state, I began the visual imagery.

I asked him to visualize an image of his colon as he imagined it would look.

"It is red, raw, and has ulcers scattered throughout," he stated.

Asking him to hold that image firmly in his mind, I then requested his patience as we began a magical, and, what may seem peculiar, conversation with his colon. "Ask your colon," I stated, "what it needs to tell you."

After several minutes he replied, "There is no answer."

I explained to him that talking to the colon in imagination is different from talking to a real live friend. He must wait quietly with patience, always in communion with this part of his body, awaiting the answer that may come in a verbal or nonverbal manner.

After several minutes of waiting, he stated, "It wants peace, quiet, and harmony." Anxiously, he then stated, "I am beginning to feel tense."

I asked him to stay with the feeling of tenseness and tightness and intensify it to increase his awareness of this feeling. "Ask your colon when all this tenseness began," I said.

His answer came surprisingly quickly. "Twenty five years ago."

I noted that his colon must have been very patient with him for all those years. Tearfully, he slowly began to access the important information hidden in his mind.

"We were not supposed to feel angry, express feelings, or disturb anyone. We were taught to be proper, pleasing. . . . I need to express my anger. . . . I need to be able to say no when I feel no. . . . I need to be able to express and care for my needs."

At this point, his agitation diminishing, he sighed with apparent relief, and slowly returned to a more relaxed state.

After several moments of quiet, I asked him to check with his colon to see if he had it correct.

"It says yes," he responded.

"Work out a contract with your colon," I told him, further explaining that this was a symbolic contract; a commitment to "listen" and respond to the physiologic needs of his body.

"I will work on these issues if my colon will be patient with me."

He opened his eyes, metaphorically as well as physically, and we planned the next few visits and the work ahead.

His disease could not be understood from either an exclusively physical or psychological perspective. An internist would have focused on his colon, a psychologist on his mind. Mind-body healing does not make this distinction. People do not come as parts.

John, intermittently disabled by his illness, had needed the treatment available through conventional medicine to reduce his symptoms and allow him to return to work and his daily activities. He wanted, however, more than treatment. He wanted to go beyond a reduction of his symptoms, he wanted to return to full health. As we will see later, John chose to begin a program of self-healing.

TREATMENT OR HEALING?

My medical school teachers never raised this question. I learned to treat illness: to match the right drug to a set of symptoms; to expect patients to comply with instructions and behave passively; to measure success by reduction in symptoms, results of laboratory tests, or duration of hospital stay. This was a technology of treatment using external agents or interventions, drugs, surgery, radiation, or physical therapy. There was no instruction in stress management, nutrition, or exercise— techniques for healing that use our natural capabilities; nor did it include the art of listening and learning about the individual being treated. Most notably, our instruction completely lacked any reference to the capacity of the human mind and body to self-heal.

As a young physician, I began my career at a large HMO. I soon became proficient at seeing many patients each day. As I gained experience practicing medicine, I discovered that conventional treatment, what I was taught in medical school, was ineffective at permanently relieving the symptoms I was treating. My patients were frequently returning with the same or related problems, most often resulting from stress and unhealthy life-styles. After several years, I began to feel overwhelmed, stressed, and fatigued from practicing a treatment-oriented medicine that was working for neither my patients nor myself. So, I began to explore alternatives to the treatment model and soon discovered that treatment and healing were not the same. Attempting to sort through these issues, I began by clarifying the difference between the two approaches.

Treatment is the use of an outside agent, or power, usually in the form of medication, surgery, radiation, or physical therapy, to manipulate the physical body with the goal of reducing or eliminating the signs and symptoms of disease. Healing is the use of the inner power and resources of our mind and body to restore our own unique balance and harmony. It is this balance and harmony that results in full health and gives us the ability to live lives of vitality and joy.

The sophisticated hard technology of treatment is a sharp contrast to the soft technology of mind-body healing. Consider the setting in which each occurs. Treatment is based in the doctor's office or a hospital, usually busy, loud, and intrusive environments. Healing requires solitude, a natural, comfortable, peaceful setting, and nonurgent time for self-reflection, learning, gradual change, and the experience of balance and harmony.

By emphasizing the expertise of the physician in matters pertaining to health the treatment model delegitimizes the essential role of the individual in his or her own healing. This results in the loss of self-healing skills and, even worse, a lack of awareness that there is more to health than the absence of the signs or symptoms of illness. In this manner, the treatment model may at times, in the long term, place the individual at an increased risk for illness. In contrast, the healing model views the individual as central to his or her healing, and aspires to a broader vision of health and well-being.

Treatment is expensive, invasive, and often rife with side effects that, at times, may be worse than the disease being treated. Healing requires the commitment and willingness to allocate time to oneself and to give priority to full health. It is self-directed, natural rather than imposed, and, unlike some effects of treatment, the effects of healing can only be positive.

As treatment is directed at the reduction and elimination of symptoms, and infrequently at actual cure, healing is directed at mobilizing the mind and body to enhance the natural defenses, accelerate recovery from illness, and promote full health. It is directed at the early, subtle, and fundamental sources of distress that lend themselves to self-regulation. This includes the following: 1) emotional distress resulting from unresolved and unhealthy feelings of powerlessness, deprivation, loneliness, and inadequacy and 2) unhealthy behaviors and life-styles. These early warning signs of imbalance are precursors of mind-body stress that, inevitably, when unheeded, lead to overt disease.

These are not exciting and dramatic issues that call upon trauma centers, intensive care, and the technological mastery of organ transplantation. These are soft issues that, when unabated over time, can be the cause of profound physiologic disturbances that may set the stage for the future breakthrough of illness. Yet, even though waiting until illness presents itself at a late stage is the most expensive form of medical care, crisis care continues to be our exclusive approach to health and disease.

The urgency of crisis, when illness has reached a level of severe mind-body imbalance, requires treatment. This is not a time for subtle, long-term self-healing that requires a consciousness and presence that is possible for very few individuals at a time of great pain and distress. Instead, crisis is usually a time to choose available treatment technologies and to allow a physician to assume the role of expert and, with sensitivity and skill, direct therapy for the malfunctioning organ or system until the immediate crisis is over and self-healing practices can be initiated.

The differences in these two approaches to health and disease are dramatic, and yet they are complementary:

Treatment	Healing
External manipulation	Self-regulation
Used in crisis	Long-term, continuous
Mechanistic, symptom-oriented	Holistic, system-oriented
Professional authority	Self-responsibility
Goal is the absence of signs or symptoms of disease	Goal is experiencing full health, wholeness

Expanding on treatment to include healing, shifting from professional direction to self-regulation, from an emphasis on the absence of
symptoms to a focus on full health is as revolutionary to contemporary
medicine as was the introduction of antibiotics in the 1940s. Change,
however, is certain as new research findings substantiate the age-old
knowledge of the self-healing powers of the mind and body.

THE WELLNESS AND HOLISTIC MOVEMENTS

The past two decades have produced an explosion of ideas and practices
claiming to fill the void left by the limitations of modern medicine. The
divergence of ideas at times has seemed confusing, yet, from a long
perspective, they contribute to the emergence of a new model for health
and healing.

For example, in the late 1970s, John Travis opened the first wellness
center in Mill Valley, California. His inspiration came from a book
written by Halbert Dunn in the 1950s, based on a series of radio talks,
entitled *High Level Wellness*. Travis believed wellness to be an educational process through which a committed individual could assume
personal responsibility for enhancing well-being. Wellness was not the
absence of illness but the presence of happiness, purpose in life, satisfying work, joyful relationships, a healthy body and living environment.

This idea of getting educated for one's own health caught on with the
general public, who saw an alternative to the traditional medical
model, which neither included a role for personal initiative, nor concerned itself with positive well-being or pro-active prevention. In the
1980s, corporations moved rapidly into wellness as a way to express
concern for their employees, boost morale, potentially moderate the
escalating costs of health care, and reduce the costs to the employer
resulting from poor employee fitness and its effect on absenteeism,
disability, worker turnover, and productivity.

Hospitals, too, entered the wellness business to enhance their public
image and diversify their sources of income. Fitness centers, health-food
stores, and an endless series of books and audio- and videotapes com-
pete for a percentage of this new market.

Wellness is, in fact, an established national movement. More than 50
percent of our population actively exercises, smoking has decreased in

the past three decades by 50 percent, health-food stores have expanded from twelve hundred in 1968 to eighty-three hundred in 1981, and more than five hundred major corporations offer fitness programs managed by full-time fitness directors.

In the meantime, over the past decade, in the health community, if you were not a wellness practitioner, you were probably a holistic practitioner. Holism, as a concept dates back to a 1926 book entitled *Holism and Evolution* by Jan Smuts. Smuts challenged the reductionist view of medical science, which denies the complexity and multidimensionality of the human experience. He supported the idea that the whole cannot be understood by summing up the parts.

Holism, as conventionally understood, states that mind, body, and spirit are inseparable. Holistic healing expands this perspective to include an understanding of individual's attitudes, beliefs, values, support system, and environments. Such a comprehensive understanding of the causative factors in health and disease, results in more effective healing.

Hippocrates, the father of western medicine, stated much the same in his treatise *Air, Water, and Places*. He taught his students to assess carefully their clients' living environment for an understanding of their diseases. Two-and-a-half millennia later, the noted internist, Sir William Osler, stated, "It is better to know the patient that has the disease than the disease that has the patient."

Holistic healers focus on the individual, not the disease. They listen carefully, aim for an in-depth understanding of the human lives with which they work, and enlist the individual as a partner in a healing program, which encompasses mind, body, and spirit. This approach demands of the healer that he or she be personally committed to the healing process.

How have the wellness movement and holism filled the gap left by the traditional medical care system? The answer, unfortunately, is not very well. As initially conceptualized by Travis, wellness was about personal growth and development. His focus was on generating positive attitudes, emotional well-being, healthy human relationships, community, spirituality, and joy. Poured into the funnel of our physically oriented culture, it came out as nutrition, fitness, and smoking cessation taught by exercise physiologists, nutritionists, and health educators, each trained within the constraints of their narrow specialty. The emphasis on mind and spirit, essential to the core of the wellness philosophy, was lost in its commercialization.

The implementation of holism, too, has left much to be desired. Rather than encouraging the evolution of well-trained, mature, and eclectic healers, we have many poorly and narrowly trained individuals hawking one alternative treatment program or another, which, at best, may be helpful while causing no harm and, at worst, may be dangerous.

Yet, although the response to the expanding gap in our medical treatment model has been filled by neither the wellness or holistic movements, each of these attempts to expand the conventional medical model has provided new perspectives and opened the way for the ultimate emergence of a new and credible model for health and healing. We will read about such a model in the next chapters.

Chapter 2

PSYCHONEUROIMMUNOLOGY: RECONNECTING MIND AND BODY

WHEN THE TIME has come for an idea, it cannot be suppressed. If it fails to emerge in one way, it will soon break through in another form. Rising from the disappointments of the wellness and holistic movements is a new medical field of investigation, psychoneuroimmunology (PNI). In its early stages, PNI has strong promise of providing us with a model and context for understanding the mind-body mysteries, and finally opening the possibility of an expanded approach to healing.

The term *psychoneuroimmunology* brings together the disciplines of the mind (psychology), the brain (neurology), and the natural healing system of the body (the immune system). Not long ago, this merging of what were previously unrelated disciplines was unimaginable. Now, viewed as closely interactive, these disciplines are gathered together as a funding and research unit at the National Institutes of Health.

Although the notion of mind-body unity is rooted in antiquity, until now it has remained off limits to serious scientific investigation. The

15

barrier began to crumble with the emergence of psychiatric medicine earlier this century, a discipline that gave rise to the term "psychosomatic illness," meaning that mental disorder could give rise to physical disorder. Subsequent psychosocial research investigating the relationship of emotional stress to illness advanced the idea of mind-body interaction. Today's emergence of PNI as a disciplined process of scientific inquiry further confirms the mind-body concept and gives it a credibility and acceptability that can only be achieved through the rigorous scientific process that we honor and respect in our society.

THE IMPORTANT ACCIDENTS:
THE DEVELOPMENT OF PNI

Scientific breakthroughs often result from the unexpected outcomes of experiments. One such surprise occurred when Dr. Robert Ader, an early investigator in the field of PNI, was training rats to develop an aversion to saccharine-sweetened water. He accomplished this by first feeding them the sweetened water mixed with a medicine called Cytoxan. Cytoxan has two effects: it causes severe nausea, and it suppresses the immune system. The rats learned to associate the sweetened water with the drug-induced nausea. Subsequently, when fed the saccharine water without the medication, the rats quickly developed nausea. They responded as if the medication were still present; a well-known phenomenon called behavioral conditioning. [1]

Then, strangely, the rats began to die of infectious disease. Although the rats had been expected only to develop nausea when reexposed to the saccharine-sweetened water, the unexpected happened. When the drug Cytoxan was no longer present, the rats recreated the second effect of Cytoxan, suppression of the immune system. It appeared that the rat mind could be trained by the classical psychologic technique of behavioral conditioning to alter the function of the body's most important natural defense system; a system previously thought to be uncontrolled by the mind.

The unexpected again happened to a patient who was dying from cancer, as described by physician Bruno Klopfer. [2] The patient had received all available medications and was no longer responding. When he heard of a new miracle drug Krebiozen, he requested permission to participate in the experimental drug study. Reluctantly, his physicians, who believed he had only a few days to live, gave him one dose of the medicine. To the surprise of all, he responded. The tumor rapidly shrank beyond all expectations as his vitality returned.

The patient then read news reports that detailed the ineffectiveness of this new drug. He quickly relapsed. When his physician cleverly decided to offer him a double dose of Krebiozen, again the patient unexpectedly responded with marked improvement and dramatic shrinking of his tumors. Shortly afterward, an updated news account appeared. It further reported that Krebiozen had been found to be a worthless drug. A few days later the patient reappeared at the hospital with a recurrence of large tumors. Despondent, he died several days later.

Science, with its wonderful curiosity and discipline cannot ignore unexpected occurrences. These examples of how the mind can alter the basic physiology of the body were among many pieces that led investigators to seek an answer to the question: How does the mind speak to and regulate the body, and how can we use this capacity of the brain for healing? Slowly, the story has begun to unfold.

MIND-BODY CONVERSATIONS

At this writing, we know of three communication systems—the autonomic nervous system, the central nervous system, and the neuropeptide chemical messenger system. (A possible fourth system is found in the meridian system of acupuncture, which mediates mind and body relations according to this ancient oriental theory and practice of health.)

Each of these systems provides direct and instant communication between mind and body (Figure 2-1). The brain appears to play the central administrative role in translating the content of the mind, attitude, and perceptions, into nerve impulses and biochemistry. It then communicates with the body through the nervous system, consisting of nerves extending from the brain to the remainder of the body and biochemicals that circulate throughout the body.

The *autonomic nervous system* (ANS) is composed of two types of nerves that oppose each other in their actions. One increases pulse and blood pressure, cools the skin, causes sweating, and activates the

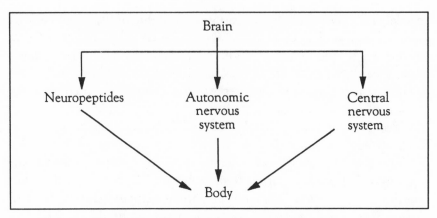

Figure 2-1. The mind-body messenger system.

production of sugar, while the other counteracts these actions by slow-ing down the body. When we are under stress, the activating aspect of this system, the sympathetic nervous system, kicks in. When we are relaxed, the quieting aspect of the system, the parasympathetic system, takes over. You can feel these systems at work when you are either agitated or at rest. The autonomic nervous system communicates the presence of stress to the body and prepares it to react to danger.

The *central nervous system* (CNS), the nerve connections that run from the brain to the body, is an important link between mind and body. It translates the intention to move a muscle into the electrical nerve impulses that result in movement of our arms and legs. Our capacity to walk, talk, and perform all of our gross and fine muscular movements results from this communication system. In the future we may discover that this system, connected by nerves to the thymus gland, spleen, and possibly other lymphatic tissue, may also play an important role in regulating the immune system. At present, there is little more to say about its role as a mind-brain messenger.

The *neuropeptide chemical messenger system* is the most recently dis-covered system that connects mind and body. When Dr. Candace Pert, working in her laboratory at Johns Hopkins University, was looking for the specific cells in the brain that are the sites of action of the opiate chemicals morphine and heroin, she found the cells to which opiates attached themselves like "a key fits a lock."[3]

Having discovered the brain cell receptors for the opiates, chemicals manufactured in test tubes and not in the body, she reasoned that the presence of these receptors must indicate that the body produces natural chemicals that fit into these same receptors. The first of these chemicals, called beta-endorphin, was soon discovered. Subsequently fifty to sixty similar natural chemicals were also discovered. These chemicals, each of which is active throughout the body, are called neuropeptides. *Neuro*, because they come from the brain, and *peptide* because they are composed of a string of basic amino acids called peptides.

This turned out to be only the beginning of a very exciting and still incomplete story. It was soon discovered that these chemicals, circulating in the blood stream, lock into receptors throughout the body, causing extensive physiologic changes in most, if not all, of the cells of the body, most important being the hormonal cells and the cells of our natural defense system, the immune system.

Further investigation led to the discovery that neuropeptides were produced both by brain cells and by cells throughout the body including the hormonal and immune cells. Not only is the brain, through the neuropeptides, able to communicate directly with the body, activating the immune and hormonal systems, but the body, by producing these same chemicals, is able to communicate back to the brain, activating the brain cells (Figure 2-2).

The immune cells are the natural defense system of the body. They maintain physiologic balance by defending against foreign invaders and repairing damage to the body. The hormonal system, using intermediary neuropeptides, called hormones, similarly maintains physiologic balance by maintaining a steady-state environment in the body

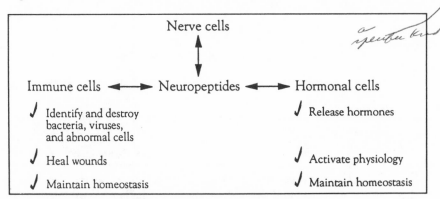

Figure 2-2. The neuropeptide system.

(homeostasis). What is unfolding is an extraordinary intercommunication system between brain and body that compels us to now view the brain and body as a dynamic interactive network.

The final, and most exciting piece of information, is that the production of these chemicals in the brain can be turned on and off by certain mental states. For example, as shown in Figure 2.3, thoughts, feelings, and images of stress, helplessness, depression, anger, and hostility are known to affect the production of these chemicals. The same appears to be true of the opposite emotions—peace, confidence, and joy. Neuropeptide synthesis also can be affected by sleep, exercise, obesity, and what are likely to be a variety of yet-to-be discovered attitudes and actions. This final link confirms the age-old wisdom that mind and body are intimately connected and interactive. Our emotions, perceptions,

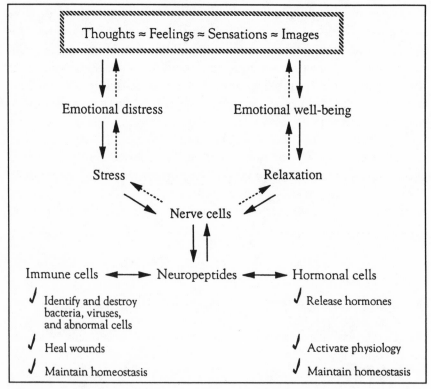

Figure 2-3. The mind-body connection. The broken arrows represent the effect on the mind of neuropeptides produced in the body. This effect has yet to be fully defined by research on PNI.

and attitudes exist not only in our mind but also are reflected in the physiology of our body. In Dr. Pert's words: "In the beginning of my work, I matter-of-factly presumed that emotions were in the head or the brain. Now I would say they are in the body as well. They are expressed in the body and are part of the body. I can no longer make a distinction between the brain and the body."[4]

The implications of these discoveries are no less than astounding. We are now confirming the capacity of the individual, through his or her attitudes and actions, to self-regulate the most minute aspects of the biochemistry and physiology of the mind and body. Applied to the immune system, this means that an individual can *choose* to either enhance or suppress it and similarly affect the function of other important physiologic systems of the body.

Beyond these implications is the important recognition that other individuals, to the extent that their attitudes and actions have a direct influence on our mental state, can also influence and control our physiology. When we become angry, stressed, feel victimized, experience joy or any other strong emotion as a direct result of our interaction with others, our physiology responds to these emotions and is thereby connected to and controlled by the attitudes and actions of the other individual. It is possible for anyone to influence directly the most minute biochemical reactions in another individual's body. This may give credence to the comment "You make me sick" and the observation that some individuals appear to be very powerful healers. The yogis, who were well aware of the vulnerability of an untrained and unsteady mind, cautioned their students to maintain a benign indifference towards those that would cause them distress and goodwill towards those who are content.

Consider further how the mental state of a powerful leader, or the imperatives of a strongly held cultural value or belief can influence the mental state and physiology of an entire group of individuals. Followed to its end, the research in PNI may well validate and amplify the discoveries of quantum physics and the metaphysical insights of the yogis; all is connected, all is interactive, all is one. It may, in fact, be true that none of us can be completely healed until we are all healed.

Scientists are now studying how this new understanding of mind-body interactiveness can be used to heal disease and promote health.

Although most of the early research is focused on disease, hopefully, future scientific research will begin to emphasize health promotion. An overview of current research includes the following:

STRESS AND IMMUNE FUNCTION

In a series of experiments on medical students, Janice K. Kiecolt-Glaser and her colleagues documented that commonplace stressful events (medical students taking examinations) resulted in immune suppression as detected in students' blood samples taken during examinations as compared to similar samples taken one month previously.[5] These effects were more marked in students whose lives were lonelier when compared with their medical school colleagues. Although these students have successfully taken examinations for many years, test taking with its fears and anxieties was still capable of affecting the immune system, as well as, we presume, other body systems.

JOB STRAIN

In a recent article, Peter L. Schnall, M.D., and his colleagues reported in JAMA on the effects of job strain on blood pressure and the heart.[6] Job strain was defined as a highly demanding job with little perceived control by the employee. They studied 215 men without evidence of coronary heart disease at seven worksites. Adjusting their study for all other related variables, they determined that individuals with job strain had a three-times higher risk of developing high blood pressure and a substantially increased incidence of structural damage to the heart. An editorial in JAMA stated, "If these results are considered along with the growing contributions of neuroscience to our understanding of how the brain speaks to the body's organs, perhaps the idea that the brain plays a role in physical disease will soon seem less 'revolutionary' and more 'normal science'."

LONELINESS AND LOSS

There are a variety of studies that document the relationship of loneliness and loss to disease. Steven Schleiffer and his colleagues at the Mount Sinai School of Medicine in New York City documented that men whose wives had recently died had a detectable suppression of the immune system during the bereavement period.[7] Several researchers have reported a higher incidence of physical and emotional disorders, including infectious disease, heart disease, and cancer, associated with marital disruption from separation and divorce. Janice Kiecolt-Glaser found depressed immune function in women separated one year or less when compared to well-matched married community counterparts.[8] Other studies indicate that poor marital quality also appears to influence health.

CARDIAC ARRHYTHMIAS

To explore the possibility that the mind could control dangerous heart arrhythmias, researchers used biofeedback equipment and a computerized electrocardiogram system to provide individuals rapid feedback of the heart rhythm. Using internal mental cues, likely mental imagery, these individuals were taught to maintain their heart rate within a narrow range and turn premature and abnormal beats on or off at will. When taken off the machines they continued to retain the capacity to control their heart rhythm.

EMOTIONAL STRESS AND INFECTION

It is considered common sense to realize that stress can make you sick. Using the herpes virus as an example, scientific research has confirmed the truth of this widely held belief. The scientific evidence for this connection has been reviewed by Janice Kiecolt-Glaser and Ronald Glaser in the November 1988 issue of *American Psychologist.*[9] Individuals exposed to this virus remain infected for their entire lifetime. The activity of the virus, whether it remains dormant or active, is thought to be directly related to the competence of the immune system. Its activity has also been shown to be related to unhappiness, stress, test taking by medical students, and recent marital disruption. Some of these effects have been shown to be reversed by relaxation interventions.

As we review this and other research it is important to remember that PNI is a new field of scientific inquiry. Scientific knowledge is not a linear process. There are some discoveries that survive and others that do not survive further examination and research. Slowly, information accumulates that has been verified and re-verified through the rigorous process of scientific research. This may take many years of hard work.

Scientists are hesitant and often unwilling to extend their findings beyond the specific circumstances and data of their studies. They well know that what may appear a logical conclusion one day, can appear different the next. This attitude is appropriate and necessary for their purposes. For those of us who care for individuals who are unable to wait until perfect clarity has been achieved, it becomes necessary and appropriate to carefully and cautiously interpret research in the context of clinical experience and information and findings from other sources. For example, it is possible and necessary for us to act on the knowledge that the mind plays a central role in the development and healing of illness before all the research is in. We can do so because we see it happening each day right in our offices, observe it in our own lives, and further support our conclusions by drawing upon research done by social scientists, psychologists and, of course, the ancient yogis. So although we must proceed, we do so with caution, anxiously awaiting for the research process to catch up, and recognizing the necessary imperfection of our knowledge and actions.

REVISITING JOHN

Let us now consider how the mind and body interact in a specific case. When John, whom I described in chapter 1, visited my office, he had already received the best that modern medicine had to offer in its treatment of ulcerative colitis. His physicians learned in their training that this disease, of unknown cause, is marked by an inflamed and ulcerated colon. They used the best available medicines to reduce the severe symptoms of this debilitating disease. The purpose of treatment is to reduce the inflammation. Traditional medical training does not go beyond this physically based understanding and treatment.

The mind-body perspective, on the other hand, views the physical aspects of disease as the obvious part of a more complex process. With John, in order to uncover the subtle aspects of his disease, it was necessary for me to use his physical symptoms as a key to information stored deeper in less accessible parts of his memory. Using a relaxation technique to quiet his mind and diminish any fear and defensiveness, he was able to bring to his awareness emotions and important aspects of his history that were central to his understanding of his disorder.

With experience, I have learned to watch carefully and patiently for information that can arise subtly either verbally or nonverbally. I have also learned to observe the sequence in which the information emerges. John first expressed sadness, then anxiety, and then anger. He expressed each of these states both emotionally and physically. Working further, we uncovered additional feelings of helplessness and powerlessness associated with an early childhood trauma: the inability to express anger.

Here, then, was the key. John, knowing he was not permitted to express strong feelings of anger, repeatedly did the only thing he could: he kept the anger, helplessness, powerlessness, and resultant anxiety and despondence inside. Although we are getting ahead of our story, it is important to know that, according to current research in PNI, feelings such as these cause the brain to communicate with the body and direct it to alter its biochemistry to a pattern that reflects in the body the mental stress in the mind. Among these changes, the pulse and blood pressure increase, muscles tighten, blood shifts from the skin to the internal organs, biochemical changes occur on the cellular level, and, most important, the immune system is suppressed.

When John was forced to contain his angry feelings as a child, the associated emotional and biochemical changes were recorded and stored in his memory. This is called state-dependent learning. Later, whenever confronted with a similar situation, his memory file unlocked and called up the response. John's entire file opened, and he would be swept, mind and body, back to this learned mind-body state. We all know the feeling of being caught up in intense emotions that seem to overwhelm us.

In further interviews with John, I learned that, in the year preceding the onset of colitis, he was involved in a relationship with a woman who, not surprisingly, resembled his mother in her discomfort with, and disapproval of, his emotions. The more he attempted to express his intense feelings, the more she withdrew. He was forced to keep his feelings inside or lose the relationship. He felt trapped and helpless.

For at least one year John activated the memory file. He experienced anger, anxiety, helplessness, and all of the associated biochemical changes, including immune system suppression. It was within this context that John developed ulcerative colitis. His physicians only saw the label; they never opened the file. The symptoms of colitis could be suppressed with medicines, but, for healing to take place, the deeper wounds had to be addressed.

Using John as an example, Figure 2.4 outlines how the mind-body system works. There is a continuous chain of events that begins with his fear of disapproval (this fear is a result of his early childhood experiences, which color and intensify his interpretations and reactions to his girlfriend's behavior) and ultimately results in overt disease. By understanding the sources of John's disease, it becomes possible to shift from treatment to healing.

THE NEED FOR NEW DEFINITIONS

By accepting that the mind and body function as a single, undivided, living unit, we can begin to move beyond treatment to healing. This shift creates a significant problem with language. The words mind and body connote two distinct objects or ideas. Although from a metaphysical or parapsychologic perspective, some may distinguish mind and body as separate, in our daily lives, they can be considered as inseparably interactive. However difficult it is to incorporate this radical idea into our thinking, we have no choice but to begin. I ask the reader to bear with my use of the word mind-body, and understand that it means the undivided functional unity through which we express our daily lives.

John and I were forced to work with these language difficulties as I interpreted for him my assessment of the ulcerative colitis as a mind-body problem. Although John had sensed his problem to be more complex than the appearance of inflammation and ulcers in his colon, and intuitively believed healing was possible, it was difficult to move away from the questions: Did my mind cause it? Can I cure my colon? Finally, we took the first step toward understanding each other, and could move forward to outline a mind-body approach to healing.

We started talking about stress. Stress, I explained to him, has three components: 1) the event that appears to trigger the problem, 2) the personality that responds with distress, and 3) the coping skills available to the individual. Given a situation, ten people would respond ten different ways. It is the uniqueness of our personalities, attitudes, and

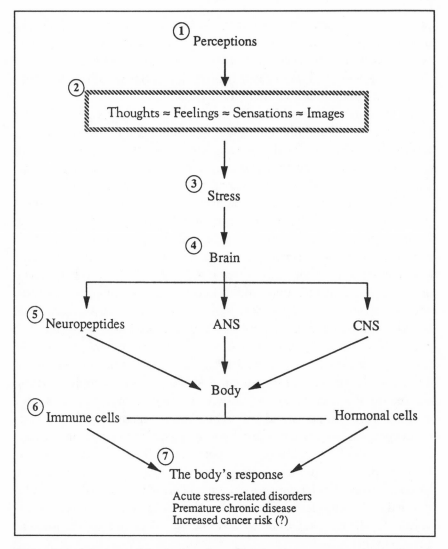

Figure 2-4. John's mind-body disorder. ① John perceives that his girlfriend disapproves of the expression of his feelings of anger. ② This results in John suppressing his anger and revisiting his old thoughts, feelings, images, and bodily sensations that are contained in his memory file, "expressing emotions results in disapproval." ③ This results in inner conflict and emotional distress. ④ The brain, responding to emotional stress, activates the mind-brain communications system. ⑤ The messengers inform the body of the emotional stress. ⑥ The immune, hormonal, and other body systems shift and respond to the state of stress. ⑦ These changes place John at risk for a variety of disorders.

perspectives that determines our reaction to a situation. Similarly our unique support systems determine how much stress we can handle before discomfort becomes distress. Once the brain senses distress, it directs the body to shift its biochemistry. John's healing program would have to work with each of these aspects of stress.

My recommendations to John began with the suggestion that he move away from his daily life for two weeks and spend that time eating well and relaxing at a health retreat. Upon his return we would begin with a relaxation training program, a progressive exercise program, dietary changes, and weekly sessions to explore through dialogue and mindfulness training (a technique described in the following chapter) his manner of working with anger, and his difficulty in sustaining healthy intimate relationships. Learning about the personal cost of his retained childhood patterns will enable him to move beyond this stage of his life into his adult years where it is possible for him to learn to be assertive, to express feelings, and to live with a sense of personal power and effectiveness. As we worked with this program, I assured him we would continue his medications to relieve the disabling symptoms.

Next we discussed our respective roles in John's healing process. My role was to assist him in understanding the nature of his disease and to develop with him a healing program. I would also assist him in learning the techniques and practices essential to his program. Throughout, I would serve as a support and, when needed, as an advisor. His role was to accept complete responsibility for how he used the knowledge he now had and would be gaining. The persistent effort to move through frustration, boredom, and, at times, skepticism was a contribution only he could make. Under conventional medical treatment, John could be satisfied with limited results and taking direction from a medical professional. Healing called John to a deeper involvement in his life, far beyond an office visit.

In the past few years, many changes have taken place in John's life. Recently, he moved to another part of the country and wrote to me to relate his progress. The following excerpt from his letter shows how the focus of John's life has moved from illness to full health:

> I am realizing how joy is found not only in myself but in every other person, and this leads to the beautiful feeling of wholeness, of which I am just beginning to see glimpses. I love the feeling of my new-found

balance and to know that peace and joy are my right and inherent in me. How wonderful. And what a relief to know the external world has no control over me. I only have to look within for guidance.

P.S. As for the colitis, it pops up now and then which merely strengthens my healing program.

What a change. Finally, a slow but certain healing.

SELF-HEALING

The gap between conventional medical treatment and healing is closing fast. John's case history demonstrates the capacity of a committed and disciplined individual to heal his mind and body. Like John, we are discovering that we are not the helpless victims of our genetics, environment, or family history.

As the human potential movement has taught us to assume and assert control over our lives, a renewed focus on self-healing can extend this teaching to include the possibility that we can assert control over many more of the activities of our mind and body than previously considered possible. For example, we know from our studies in biofeedback that individuals can regulate finger temperature to tenths of a degree, alter electrical potentials in muscles, control brain wave activity, lower blood pressure, and decrease the pulse rate. We further know of the extraordinary physiologic control that yogis can exert. Now we are discovering the whys and hows from our scientists. As we assume this control, we take ownership of our personal power.

The research in PNI and other important advances are forging the important links between mind and body, expanding the frontiers of healing. To use this new knowledge to our advantage, we must understand and assert control over our minds and bodies. The next two chapters present the two components of self-healing: mindfulness and self-regulation. Mastering these two techniques can assist you in moving beyond treatment to healing and full health.

Chapter 3

MINDFULNESS

IN THE LAST chapter, we learned that PNI is confirming it is possible to self-regulate many, if not all, of the functions of our minds and bodies. There are many implications to this discovery. Foremost is the emerging recognition that each of us possesses a natural capacity for self-healing, the capacity to restore wholeness and balance in our lives. Healing has two components: mindfulness and self-regulation, shown in Figure 3.1.

These two components, mindfulness and self-regulation, can be viewed as corresponding to the two major components of conventional medical treatment, diagnosis and therapy. Mindfulness and self-

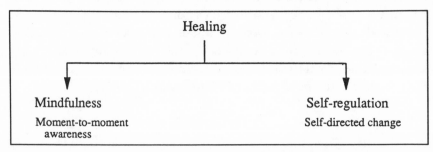

Figure 3-1. The two components of healing.

regulation are directed toward health promotion and primary prevention, and diagnosis and therapy are exclusively directed toward the elimination or lessening of disease. This chapter introduces the first component of healing: mindfulness.

THE WORKINGS OF THE MIND

To understand mindfulness, we need to know more about how the mind works. The mind has two basic activities or operating systems. The first is "mind-talk." The second is what we will call "mindfulness." These two activities of the mind, mind-talk and mindfulness, cannot occur simultaneously. Either one or the other is active at any moment. Mind-talk is the usual mental chatter. It is the predominant automatic activity of the mind. Mindfulness is a chosen and self-initiated activity of the mind. It does not happen automatically or naturally. It requires conscious effort.

Mind-talk has four aspects: thoughts, feelings, images, and sensations. One or more of these aspects may be active at any one moment. Mindfulness consists of three aspects: attention, concentration, and meditation. These aspects occur sequentially: attention precedes concentration, which precedes meditation. These are shown in Figure 3.2.

Mind-talk, the predominant activity of the mind, is the end result of the interaction of our sensory system with the outer world. The sensory system, a specialized part of the brain, records and transmits to awareness the experience of sight, sound, smell, taste, and touch. It is the

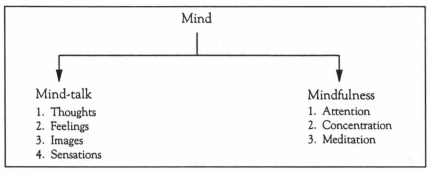

Figure 3-2. The activities of the mind.

intermediary between ourselves and everything outside of us, making it possible for us to experience and know the outer world. As illustrated in Figure 3.3, from the earliest moments in life, each individual we meet and each experience we have is taken in through these senses. The accumulated pieces of information are stored in the brain as memories (memories can be understood as the "footprints" left by prior life experiences). The brain files this information in two basic categories: factual and psychologic information.

Factual information helps us to move through daily life. It provides us with instant access to knowledge about objects and places. It is the kind of information we learn in school. Psychologic information is more subjective. It consists of our impressions, perceptions, and interpretations of our personal experiences. It is usually learned through our interactions with others. It defines our self-image and the manner in which we relate to the outer world. Both kinds of information can remain dormant and inactive or can be activated by events and circumstances that unlock our memory. The continuous activation and recollection of both factual and psychologic information and the associated thoughts, feelings, images, and sensations is the mental activity we call mind-talk.

Recalling factual information is usually, but not always, helpful. For example, it allows us to do our work efficiently, make the correct turns when driving home in the evening, and automatically use modern sophisticated devices. At other times, when used without mindfulness

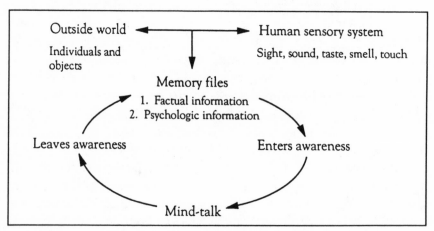

Figure 3-3. The development of mind-talk.

and care, it can be quite destructive as with the use of our sophisticated technology to develop nuclear weapons, or the destruction of our environment due to careless industrialization.

Psychologic information can be healthy or unhealthy. Unhealthy psychologic information is invariably false and inaccurate information most often resulting from a young child's mistaken interpretations of his or her early life experiences. As an example, parents, because of their personal discomfort with conflict and anger, may discourage and shut-off the expression of anger by their child. The child learns and carries into adulthood the misperception that expressing anger is an inappropriate response with negative consequences. This misinformation can destroy adult relationships, resulting in unnecessary pain and suffering. In contrast, healthy psychologic information results from life experiences that support healthy emotional development. This information causes neither pain nor suffering. It leads to the development of healthy attitudes, actions, and life-styles.

Mind-talk relies on stored information. It is always a recollection from the past. Our past experiences program our brain much as a computer is programmed by a programmer. The automatic, uncontrolled, unconscious, unchanging, and mechanical output of the brain is experienced as mind-talk. When our mind is engrossed in mind-talk we forget the present moment and become absorbed in memory. We cannot fully hear another individual when our mind is talking about work. We cannot experience the beauty of a walk in nature when we are focused on financial worries, nor can we appreciate the growing experiences of our children when distracted by other matters. The more aware we become of mind-talk, the more we realize how little we attend to the present moment—the only experience that is actually happening at that time. Our constant absorption in mind-talk deadens our lives as we unconsciously carry forth the conventions and customs of our families and cultures with little awareness of who and what we are, separate from what we have learned and gathered from others and society.

Fortunately, the mind has another activity: mindfulness. When we shift from an absorption in mind-talk to an attention to the present moment we begin to remember where we are, who we are, and what is happening now. This is mindfulness, the important, and, for many, unknown, activity of the mind that can wake us from our "sleep" and allow us to experience and participate in the pulsating, ever-changing, sensuous vitality of the here and now.

Mindfulness reveals itself when mind-talk has ceased to occupy our awareness automatically and unconsciously. It is a precise, direct, ongoing observation of our inner and outer experiences as they are occurring in the here and now. This may be an important work project, a conversation, a meal, driving on the freeway, or even mind-talk (there is a difference between observing mind-talk and being absorbed in it). Mindfulness is a consciously chosen, deliberate attention to the present moment experience. It is chosen only by those who know the difference between being asleep and being awake, both in the figurative sense. When the mechanical mind takes over, and we automatically return to mind-talk, we can choose to intervene and shift our attention back to the present moment. An individual's capacity for mindfulness can range from the blindness of a Willy Loman in *Death of a Salesman*, who is lost in his fantasized inner dialogue, to the finely tuned mindfulness of a yogi or zen master.

Mindfulness experiences the present moment without reference to the past. Once we begin to evaluate, judge, review, or conceptualize, we are no longer mindful, but rather in the process of storing the present moment into memory and creating future mind-talk. Mindfulness, which focuses exclusively on the present moment, exists outside of time. It is the presence and complete attention that every individual experiences at one time or another when reading a book, immersing oneself in a creative act, experiencing the solitude of nature, or being fully present with another person. At moments such as these, moments of flow, there is no time, hours can seem like seconds. For however briefly, we have experienced the timelessness and vitality of mindfulness.

Mindfulness works with our busyness, restlessness, anxiety, urgency, and compulsiveness, all of which come from past fears and conditioned imperatives expressed through mind-talk. It allows us to settle down, to quiet, to see and experience what is happening in our lives in contrast to what is happening in our minds. It has three aspects: attention, concentration, and meditation. Each is important to learn and understand.

Attention is the continuous uninterrupted experience of a chosen object of attention. Anything can serve as focal point: a physical object, an individual, an activity, our body, mind, deeper self, or the various experiences that are ongoing in any moment in our lives. Attention occurs when we begin to observe our experiences rather than moving through life asleep. When we brush our teeth we know we are brushing our teeth, when we are walking we know we are walking. We are aware of the sensations and the experiences of life in contrast to the stored memories in our brain.

Attention allows us to be aware of and experience, without interpretations, judgments, and the distortions of mind-talk, the present moment. It is quite difficult to remain mindful and attentive for more than a few seconds. Try it. Take a break in your reading and focus on an object in front of you. See how long you can hold the focus without the intrusion of mind-talk. If you are distracted, return to your focus and attempt to hold it as long as possible. If you can hold attention long enough, you may feel a sense of calmness moving through your body, and your experience of the object may shift, change, and deepen. Continue this, if possible, for two minutes. If you have courage, see how long you can be aware of your experiences today. You will likely discover that, irrespective of your sincere efforts, you wake-up halfway through the day recognizing that you have forgotten yourself most of the day.

If you are able to maintain and hold attention without distraction, you will shift into concentration, the second aspect of mindfulness. Concentration differs from attention. With practice, it allows your awareness to penetrate the surface characteristics of the object of your attention and to experience a more comprehensive, unchanging, and fundamental understanding of its essential nature in contrast to the limited understanding that is based on superficial appearance. The former cannot be achieved through an intellectual process that emphasizes analytic thinking. It requires mindfulness. We will return to concentration and learn how to use it in this way in chapter 7.

With practice it becomes possible to sustain attention and concentration for extended periods of time. The mind quiets and mind-talk ceases to preoccupy us. What remains is only the object of attention, the experience of the moment. If you choose to enter the meditative state, slowly the object moves out of awareness and what remains is an empty mind. This begins the third aspect of mindfulness, meditation. Meditation is characterized by feelings of clarity, tranquility, and peace. It occurs when the movement of the mind, mind-talk, is finally arrested through attention and concentration. What is experienced at this point is so subtle that it is difficult to convey with words. The mind finally rests in silence: the peace of meditation. We become aware of the empty mind, the mind without cognitions, what some call the "original mind." There is a nonselective and comprehensive awareness of inner and outer experiences that has been called "choiceless awareness." The poets express it best:

At the still point of the turning world. Neither flesh nor fleshless:
Neither from nor towards; at the still point, there the dance is,
But neither arrest nor movement. And do not call it fixity,
Where past and future are gathered. Neither the movement
       from nor towards,
Neither ascent nor decline. Except for that point, the still point,
There would be no dance, and there is only the dance.
I can only say there we have been: I cannot say where.
And I cannot say, how long, for that is to place it in time.

T. S. ELIOT
The Four Quartets

. . . a sense sublime
Of something far more deeply interfused,
Whose dwelling is the light of setting suns,
And the round ocean and the living air,
And the blue sky, and in the mind of man;
A motion and spirit, that impels
All thinking things, all objects of all thought,
And rolls through all things.

WILLIAM WORDSWORTH
Tintern Abbey

QUICK RECAP

Activities	Mind-talk	Mindfulness
Aspects	Thinking	Attention
	Sensing	Concentration
	Imaging	Meditation
	Feeling	
Characteristics	Scattered thinking	Focused awareness
	Restless mind	Quiet mind
	Activated body	Still body
Sources	Memory	Present moment
	Current events	

Table 3-1. How the mind works

Learning to quiet the automatic and mechanical mind of mind-talk and shift to mindfulness is the essential first step in healing. It is through attention, concentration, and meditation that we can develop an accurate and precise awareness of our minds, bodies, and outer world, an awareness that is essential for full health.

DEVELOPING MINDFULNESS

Recent years have provided us with an increased exposure to Eastern philosophy and mindfulness practices. From these we have gained the opportunity to learn and expand upon the simple yet extraordinary techniques for achieving mindfulness. The goals of these practices are 1) achieving self-understanding and insight, which is arrived at through training the mind for precise and sensitive self-observation, and 2) cultivating the peaceful and silent mind, which is arrived at through the persistent practice of meditation.

There are two ways to develop mindfulness: 1) practicing mindfulness in our daily lives and 2) regular practice of a mindfulness training exercise. In our daily lives we can either live automatically, half-asleep with little awareness, or we can choose to be aware of what is happening. Each activity, big or small, is an opportunity to practice mindfulness. If your time for structured mindfulness training is limited, use your life. Tap yourself on the shoulder to wake-up. If you are listening to the radio, listen to the radio, if you are talking on the phone, attend to the conversation, if you are walking, know you are walking. Each time you remember who you are, where you are, and what is happening you are training yourself in mindfulness, and experiencing one more moment of aliveness.

The second and complementary approach to mindfulness training requires a daily structured training session. Before going further and considering the mindfulness training exercises, it is valuable to consider three important elements of mindfulness training: attitude, solitude, and patience.

ATTITUDE

A certain attitude is necessary before you attempt to learn mindfulness. You must be committed and strongly motivated to move beyond a surface understanding of distress to full health. Because healing is a long-term, continuous investment in achieving and maintaining full health, mindfulness requires dedicated time and effort. There will be many moments of doubt, frustration, indecision, and boredom that can only be traversed with faith in your long-term goal and persistence in getting there. Healing is far different from a brief symptom-oriented encounter in a medical office.

In the beginning, most individuals undertake mindfulness training to assist with a difficult problem, often stress, which has been unresponsive to other approaches and is unacceptably disruptive to daily life. With time and effort, the individual begins to understand the role of mindfulness in improving the quality of life and enhancing health. The mind stays quieter, relationships are easier, overreaction to difficult situations decreases, insight and understanding matures, and, for brief moments, there is serenity and peace. In time, effort seems less necessary as an increasing understanding of the value of mindfulness draws the individual towards a new way of living. Mindfulness slowly becomes the norm.

SOLITUDE

Solitude is the second essential consideration in learning mindfulness. It removes us from the everyday world and creates a supportive environment for learning and practicing mindfulness. Creating quiet time in the modern world is not easy, however. Life as we live it today does not cooperate with our need for solitude. It is filled with distractions that encourage mind-talk. The telephone, car radio, beeper, and other endless sounds of activity seem to be everywhere.

It is difficult to determine what purpose is served by all the noise in our lives. For some, silence may even feel disorienting and unfamiliar. The automatic response is to turn again to distractions such as the radio, TV, or idle conversation. For others, solitude gives rise to unpleasant feelings of loneliness, feelings that should be explored and understood rather than avoided. Still others associate endless activity and sensory stimulation with being alive. When things quiet down, new distractions must be found to avoid the emptiness of solitude.

Certainly, some important experiences are facilitated by our interactions with other people. These include companionship, physical and emotional intimacy, and shared support. Other experiences, however, are nurtured by solitude. These include creativity, insight, self-discovery, spirituality, and inner harmony and balance. These experiences that are nurtured by solitude can all be consequences of the practice of mindfulness; a practice that requires a personal concern for solitude and silence.

Mindfulness training requires removing yourself from outside activities for solitude at least one hour each day, and, occasionally, for a longer personal retreat. For some this may be time for a walk, exercise, listening to music, or quiet reading. A portion of this time, thirty minutes each day, should be used for mindfulness training.

To the novice, the usual response to such a suggestion is: "I don't have time to sit and do nothing when I have such an active schedule, maybe next week." More mind-talk. However, "nothing"—meaning the absence of outside "productive" activities—is essential for healing. It forces us to look beyond our culturally conditioned view of what is valuable. What is happening may seem like nothing, but inside, the stillness leads to mental clarity, insight, relaxation, and physiologic healing. Treatment requires time at the physician's office, completing examinations, and following a treatment program until the signs and symptoms are gone. Healing requires a long-term commitment to spending time with yourself. It is something no one tells us to do. We must choose it ourselves.

We all have daily lives that are filled with important responsibilities. For some of us, at one time or another in our lives, our days are overfilled with unchangeable responsibilities such as child care or the need to work long hours to earn a living. Although it may be difficult to set aside specific time for mindfulness training, it may be possible to 1) increase "quiet time" by reducing unnecessary noise and distraction, 2) maximize shorter periods of mindfulness training, 3) use ordinary and everyday life experiences for practicing mindfulness, and 4) practice the breathing exercises described in the later chapters, which require less time and less emphasis on solitude. In this manner, even the busiest individual can begin a self-healing program now.

PATIENCE

Patience is the third element of mindfulness training. Just as years of learning cannot be undone in hours, the skills and self-knowledge that are required for mindfulness and self-regulation are acquired over many years. These result from a conscious and mindful approach to life, and a committed process of self-inquiry. Life becomes a daily movement toward health, peace, love, and joy. It is an experience to be lived, not a problem to be solved. Patience is essential for self-healing.

We must be like the young child learning to walk for the first time. Each time he falls he gets up again. He never doubts his capacity to walk, never stops getting up and advancing his skill. He is persistent and clear about his goal, enjoying most, if not all of the moments of the process. If we approached learning to walk the way most of us approach our health, we would still be crawling. Take your time, enjoy it, be patient, and do not forget to get up when you fall.

These elements—attitude, solitude, and patience—are the keys to mindfulness training. They provide the context within which it is possible to retrain the mind and shift it from its predominant adult activity, mind-talk, to mindfulness. The following exercises will assist you in beginning your study and practice of mindfulness.

INTRODUCTION TO THE EXERCISES

This and the following chapters present a variety of exercises designed to amplify the text and provide you with a direct experience of the ideas and concepts described here. With the exception of the mindfulness training exercise, which requires daily practice, all other exercises should be practiced in conjunction with the corresponding text. These exercises can and should be repeated as many times as necessary to maximize the understanding of the text.

The exercises can be practiced in pairs with individuals taking turns reading to each other, or you can record them on an audiocassette and play them back to yourself. You will notice that, in the text of the exercises, I have frequently added dialogue that expands upon or reviews the previously presented concepts. For some individuals, listening to such information can be an important supplement to reading it. Because this is the way I use these exercises in my practice, I suggest that the added dialogue be recorded with the remainder of the exercise and listened to with closed eyes.

Note that the time for pauses is suggested in parenthesis. If you are recording the exercise, simply remain silent for the indicated time. Also, when reading the exercises, allow pauses between sentences to permit for the responses to instructions within paragraphs.

EXERCISES FOR LEARNING MINDFULNESS

Learning mindfulness requires: 1) the daily practice of the mindfulness training exercise (to be introduced later in this chapter) and 2) the use of mindfulness in the activities of daily living. In the following exercises you will experience each of these steps.

First, you will focus on directly experiencing and observing your personal mind-talk. Next, you will observe how your mind moves from mind-talk and its four aspects—thoughts, feelings, images, and sensations—to mindfulness and its three aspects—attention, concentration, and meditation—and, unfortunately, how it too frequently returns again to mind-talk. You will notice how mind-talk is the dominant activity of the mind—always pulling the mind in its direction, away from mindfulness. You will also notice the intense effort that is initially necessary to focus the mind for even a few moments. The final exercises in this chapter will assist you in practicing mindfulness in daily life. I suspect that, as you work with these exercises and those in the other chapters, you will begin to glimpse, and then experience for longer periods, the understanding, peace, and joy of the mindful state so important to the healing process.

EXERCISE 1:
_____

MIND-TALK

Assume a comfortable position and close your eyes. The intent of this exercise is to give you direct experience with the first of the two activities of the mind: mind-talk. If you personally explore and directly discover how your mind works you will understand it and more effectively use the information presented.

Mind-talk is one of the two ways in which the mind works. In the untrained mind, mind-talk is the predominant activity. It is an automatic and mechanical process, an unceasing flow. It continuously rambles, bringing to awareness fragments of information that relate to current events, past experiences, or thought patterns that have been stored away in the mind. Mind-talk has only four ways of expressing itself: thoughts, feelings, images, and sensations.

Now, become aware of any thoughts as they enter your mind. Thoughts about yesterday, today, this exercise, or this book. Thoughts relating to personal concerns, desires, worries, hopes, fears. Listen carefully, imagine that you are about to hear important information. Observe your mind with the detachment of a journalist. Be receptive and alert. (pause three minutes)

Notice how thoughts arise. Become aware of how one thought gives rise to another thought and then another. (pause one minute) Notice how a thought may lead to a feeling, sensation, or image. (pause one minute) Notice how thoughts demand your attention, urging you to attend to and analyze them. (pause one minute) They act like a strong magnet drawing you tightly to them. Not infrequently, an extended internal dialogue may begin as if two or more persons were engaged in a lively conversation. You may discover yourself completely absorbed and oblivious to experiences that are occurring in the moment. Continue to observe your mind-talk. (pause three minutes)

Now we will experiment with mind-talk. As you become aware of the thoughts, label them: past, present, future, worries, judgments, fears, likes, dislikes, or future plans. (pause two minutes)

Next begin to count the different thoughts that move in and out of your mind. See how many thoughts you can count in the next minute. (pause one minute)

Next, draw your attention to your breath. Become aware of its movement in and out through your nostrils. Count how long you can maintain this focus before you are distracted by a thought. Try this several times and see if you can discover who is in charge of your consciousness; you or your automatic mind. (pause two minutes)

Leaving thoughts behind, redirect your attention to any feelings you are currently experiencing. (pause one minute) As before, allow your feelings to freely enter and leave your awareness. At first you may have difficulty distinguishing between your thoughts about your feelings and the feelings themselves. Feelings are felt more in the heart, the thoughts more in the mind. Some of us predominantly generate thoughts, others feelings. If, during this exercise, you discover that you are more a "thinker" than a "feeler" continue to follow the exercise working with your thoughts.

Notice the feelings. Label them: fears, worries, delight, sadness, boredom, frustration, love, dislike, envy, joy, anger, hostility, communion. (pause one minute) Watch them as they move in and out. Are they associated with thoughts? Are you compelled to analyze them? Does one feeling lead to another? Is your awareness increasingly drawn to these feelings? Do some specific feelings pull more than others? Can you observe how feelings move in and out of your awareness only to be replaced by others? Does your body react to these feelings? (pause three minutes)

Leaving your feelings, let us now move to the many sensations that can arise spontaneously in your mind. Are you experiencing warmth or coolness? (pause thirty seconds) Are you hearing external sounds? Are you aware of smells? (pause thirty seconds) Is there discomfort in your body? Where is it and how intense is it? (pause thirty seconds) As with your feelings and thoughts, notice how sensations can enter awareness and leave. Notice how they can be associated with feelings and thoughts. Notice how your mind can become preoccupied with certain sensations. (pause one minute)

Pick the strongest sensation in your body. Now focus your attention on the movement of the breath in and out of your nostrils. Count how long you can maintain this focus without being drawn back to the sensation. Where is your freedom of thought? Who is in control, you or your automatic mind? Does your mind pull you around by your nose, leading you where it wishes to go? (pause two minutes)

Finally, draw your attention to the fourth aspect of mind-talk,

images. Not all of us create images easily. We each have a
predominant mental language. Our language may be thoughts,
feelings, or sensations instead of images. If you do not make
pictures in your mind, stay with the predominant language of
your mind, using it instead of imagery in the remainder of the
exercise.

Become aware of any images in your mind. What are these
about? Are they about present concerns, past, or future? Are
they associated with feelings, thoughts, or sensations? Notice
how they enter awareness, moving in and out. Return to your
breathing. See how long you can focus on your breathing before
you are drawn back to imagery. (pause two minutes)

Conclude this exercise by allowing your mind to again move
freely. Do you predominantly speak in thoughts, feelings, images,
or sensations? Can you control this activity of your mind and its
pull on your awareness? For how long? Notice how this activity,
mind-talk, is never in the present moment. It is always old
information. Once an experience becomes a memory file, which
can take only a few seconds, it is no longer new. Mind-talk
keeps us in the past, removed from the present moment, from
what is actually happening. Finally, notice that when we
observe the mind rather than being drawn into its talk, the
mind and body quiet, leaving us more peaceful, relaxed, and
receptive. (pause two minutes)

Slowly, at your own pace, open your eyes and reorient yourself
to the room.

This exercise can provide you with important insight into the workings of your mind. You likely will observe how repetitive, disruptive,
and out-of-control your mind can be as it unceasingly produces mind-
talk. Although this is the automatic and predominant activity of the
mind, we rarely observe it, rather, we are usually lost in it.

You next may be surprised at how quiet your mind can become.
Individuals practicing this exercise often comment on how their minds
quiet as soon as they begin to observe them and give them permission to
freely "talk". This is an important observation. Whenever your attention is focused, even if it is on mind-talk, your mind will slow down and
quiet. You may further notice that, whenever your mind quiets, everything around you also quiets.

Continue to observe your mind after the exercise and later during your routine daily activities. Extend your observations to include the remainder of your body, and events outside of you. Whatever your observations, you are learning about how your mind and body works, and, to the extent that you understand it, you can use it rather than be used by it.

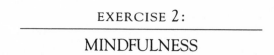

EXERCISE 2:

MINDFULNESS

This three-part exercise should be completed as one continuous exercise.

Assume a comfortable position and close your eyes. The intent of this exercise is give you direct experience with the second activity of the mind, mindfulness, and to help you explore its three components, attention, concentration, and meditation.

Remember that the mind works in two ways, mind-talk and mindfulness. Mind-talk is the predominant, automatic, and mechanical activity of the untrained mind. With training each of us can learn to shift our minds to mindfulness, the awareness of what is happening now.

The content of our mind, its thoughts, feelings, images, and sensations, is expressed through mind-talk. Mind-talk determines our mental state, shapes our physiology, and directs our day-to-day lives. It is important to understand this fact. By precisely observing our mind-talk we can learn to shut off our automatic mind and consciously choose our attitudes and actions. This is how we shift into mindfulness.

ATTENTION

The first component of mindfulness is attention. An attentive and focused mind contrasts sharply with the rambling chaotic mind of mind-talk. Attention is difficult to achieve and sustain. At one time or another, we have all experienced how it feels to be right there in the present moment. It is difficult, however, to sustain awareness of the present moment for more than four or five seconds at a time. As we train our minds to become attentive to the here and now, we can sustain attention for longer periods of time, lingering less in the distraction of mind-talk.

To train our minds in attention, we can use any object or experience. The ultimate purpose, however, is to learn to be attentive to all that is happening in each moment of our lives. In this exercise we will use the process of breathing as our focal point for training because breath is 1) always with us, 2) we can always return to it to renew our focus, and 3) ancient knowledge and modern science have affirmed the unique connection between breathing and our state of consciousness.

Begin by drawing your attention to your breath as it naturally moves in and out of your body. You may focus on 1) its movement through the nostrils, 2) the expansion and contraction of your chest, or 3) the rising and falling of your abdomen with the breathing cycle, that is, with each inhalation, your abdomen rises; with each exhalation it falls. Attempt to balance the intensity of your focus; do not force or strain, and do not hold it so loosely that your mind easily wanders. It is important that you maintain an awareness and focus on the breath. Do not mentally analyze or comment on your breathing—simply observe it.

Given the nature of your untrained mind, you may soon return to the distracting chatter of mind-talk. When this occurs, it is important to remind yourself that the purpose of this exercise is to focus your attention on what is happening in the present moment. Thus, if you notice that you are absorbed in mind-talk, a thought, feeling, sensation, or image, and are no longer focused on your breath, accept it, do not fight or resist it. Slowly shift your attention to the awareness that you are thinking, feeling, sensing, or imaging, note that that is what is happening at that moment. Observe the mind-talk—do not analyze, comment upon or become absorbed in it. It is as if you were a mountain watching clouds float overhead or a journalist carefully observing an event.

Shortly, if you continue to observe your mind rather than become absorbed by it, the mind-talk will quiet, your body will become more relaxed and you can gently return to your previous focus on the breath. If your mind returns to mind-talk again, shift your attention to observing the mind-talk; soon you can return quietly to your focus on the breath. Practice attention, the first component of mindfulness for the next ten minutes. You may find yourself commenting, judging, or analyzing during this practice. This is your mind talking again. Note it and return to your breath. (pause ten minutes)

You will notice how difficult it is to sustain your attention, and how little control you actually have over your automatic mind. Imagine what it is like when you are not even attempting to attend to the here and now. You will also notice how your automatic mind slowly begins to quiet, and, at the same time, how it subtly attempts to distract you by questioning why you are doing this and creating feelings of boredom, resistance, and frustration. Note the mind-talk and return to your breathing. You are beginning to receive the first results of attention: a clearer understanding of how your mind works.

CONCENTRATION

We are now going to shift to the second aspect of mindfulness: concentration. Concentration begins when the mind and body are quiet and still. As you are increasingly able to accomplish this, your capacity for concentration will improve.

Concentration is a shift from attention to reflection. It enables us to observe and understand further the workings of our mind and body. Because concentration is a careful, precise, and accurate process of observation, with practice we can achieve an increasingly clear and truthful understanding of ourselves, others, and ultimately the natural laws of life.

For the purpose of this exercise, and with your eyes still closed, return your focus to the breath. Observe where you best experience the movement of your breath. Is it in the area of the nostrils, chest, or abdomen? Pick whichever area you most feel your breath, and focus your attention on it. If it is the nostrils, slowly become aware of the in and out of the breath. If it is the chest or abdomen become aware of the rising of the chest and abdomen that occurs with inspiration and the falling with expiration. Continue gently noting the movement while observing your breath. (pause two minutes)

Follow your breathing closely, one breath at a time. If your mind is distracted by mind-talk, gently note this distraction to yourself and return to the breathing. If the distraction is sufficiently strong, for a few moments make this your focal point. Observe the distraction with detachment, when it quiets down return to your breathing. (two minutes)

Carefully observe the breathing process. Notice how it feels. Do you breathe predominantly through your chest or abdomen? (pause one minute) Where is the movement more pronounced? Which muscles are involved? (pause one minute) Is the quality of your breath smooth or rough? Are the other muscles of your body relaxed or tense? Check them, and, if they are tense, relax them. Notice the relationship between your breathing and the quiet or restlessness of your mind. (pause one minute) Continue to observe carefully all aspects of your breathing, returning to your breath after you note any distractions. Remember, although you may be experiencing deep relaxation this is not a relaxation exercise. It is an exercise to fine-tune your powers of observation, powers that can help you investigate and understand other aspects of your mind and body. (pause five minutes)

Now remind yourself of the attention you usually give to your breathing. How much attention do you give to your mind and body, how much attention to your life? How often are you on automatic pilot, unaware of what is happening? Without precise knowledge of how things are working in our minds and bodies, we can do little to change things. For the next few minutes return to your breath, closely observing how it works. If you are bored or distracted, bring your attention back to your breath. Boredom is rarely a statement about what you are doing but usually reflects lack of attention. (pause two minutes)

To work further with concentration is to learn how to concentrate on an issue of concern, pierce through its surface to achieve a deeper understanding without intellectually analyzing it. For example, it is important for each of us to know at any moment what the central focus of our lives is, what are we meant to be doing, what is the intent and direction of our lives at this moment? For some, this may be career, and for others relationships, family, service, or personal growth. For several minutes place this issue in you mind. Ask yourself, "At this time in my life what is the central issue I must work with?" It is like planting a seed. Plant this question in your mind and allow it to develop by itself. Do not interfere with it. Just hold the question and observe what comes forth; what insights you discover. Notice how when the appropriate insight arises it will fit like a glove. (pause ten minutes)

MEDITATION

The third and concluding section of this exercise is a natural progression from the earlier sections. Meditation differs from attention and concentration because it has no external or internal object of focus and observation. Meditation is being present. It is the state of awareness that occurs when the mind is silent, and the body is still. Meditation results when mind-talk, selective attention, and concentration cease to exist. It is a sense of emptiness (often mistaken for the opposite of fullness), peace, harmony, and a soft and expansive awareness that is undistracted by mental commentary. The mind, it can be said, rests in its natural state.

Meditation is best experienced by beginning with attention to breathing as previously done. Next, shift to concentration on the breath. With focused attention and concentration on your breath, the mind will increasingly quiet. Continue your focus on the breathing.

As you focus, when distracted by mind-talk, shift your attention to it, observe it, and when it quiets, return to your breath. Practice this for the next ten minutes. During this period of time you may experience moments of meditation. Please do not seek these moments. You will not experience them if you seek them. Simply maintain the process. (pause ten minutes)

During this time you will experience, at first for only a few fleeting moments, periods of emptiness, and pure awareness. At such moments, there is no mind as we commonly know it, and thus no desires, thoughts, or cravings. All is complete, all is at peace. With practice you will be able to hold this state for longer periods of time. (pause five minutes)

You are now discovering that solitude is different than aloneness, peace different than relaxation, and contentment different from momentary pleasure. You are learning that what is important is not the outer conditions of your life, but your inner condition. It will become increasingly more difficult for you to deny your capacity to self-determine your inner condition. A ripened fruit cannot return to the unripened state. You are investigating and realizing what the ancient great teachers knew, that you have great power to self-regulate and heal your life. (pause two minutes)

It is now time to complete this exercise. Slowly, at your own pace return to the room, and, when you are ready, open your eyes.

Following the exercise, become aware of the feeling of quiet in your mind and body. (You may resist reading further as this may feel disruptive to your inner quiet. If this is so, stop now and return later.) Notice how "slowed down" you are, how sensitive and aware you are of your surroundings and of other people. Are you more peaceful? Do you need anything? Have your felt like this before? Have you observed something new about your mind and body? Become aware of what this exercise has taught you about the workings of your mind.

Although we choose a focal point, the breath, when our mind wanders we can use this opportunity to watch the moving mind and when it quiets return to the breath. If you become frustrated, annoyed, or judgmental, remember: these disabling feelings are also mind-talk and should be observed rather than acted out.

In the beginning, it may be difficult to focus and quiet the mind. You may mistakenly believe that it is necessary to force the mind to quiet. This is not the case. Although we use the breath as our focal point, what is most important is to observe whatever is happening in the moment. In this way, you will slowly discover how your mind works and how to handle distractions. This information and further training will result, with persistence and patience, in a mind whose natural direction is towards mindfulness.

TRAINING YOURSELF IN MINDFULNESS

The following exercise is the mindfulness training exercise. It should be practiced thirty minutes each day. Early in the morning, preferably before sunrise, and shortly after arising, are the best and most natural times. At this time, the mind is rested, and the world is not yet fully awake with its noises and demands. If this is not possible designate another time and place for your training sessions. The space needs little more than a chair or sitting cushion, a sense of peacefulness, and the guarantee of uninterrupted nonurgent time.

Begin by sitting in a chair, with your eyes closed, feet uncrossed, and hands resting comfortably on your thighs. Start with a brief breathing exercise. Take a deep and full breath, blow it all out, and observe the filling of your abdomen with the next breath.

Beginning with the first in-breath, count one, and with the next in-breath, count two. Continue this process until you reach ten, and then begin again. Breathe in this manner for three cycles of ten. If you miss or forget the number, return to one and begin the cycle again. After you have completed three cycles become aware of the natural movement of your breath and the rising of your abdomen with each in-breath and its falling with each out-breath.

Allow your awareness to follow this natural movement with a comfortable concentration and focus. As a novice, or during periods of stress when you are caught in the clutter of your mind, this may be difficult. It is quite normal for your untrained mind to catch on to one or more of the random thoughts, feelings, sensations, or images that move in and out of your mind. When you notice this, become aware of what is happening. If it is a thought, notice you are thinking, stand back, and watch your mind. Avoid any analysis or judgment.

As you observe your mind, it will naturally quiet. If you resist and fight your mind, it will remain restless. As you remain focused, you will slowly shift into a deeper concentration, and, at times, to meditation. (pause ten minutes)

Observe your mind without identifying with its mind-talk. Take a neutral position, noting what is happening but not reacting to the constant movements of the mind. To a novice this will seem like detachment: a disinterest in what is occurring. In actuality, it is mindfulness, a complete, undistracted presence in the activity of the moment.

As you anchor your awareness in the present moment, in the rising-falling of the abdomen, you are dampening the natural background activity of the mind. If you feel restless, bored, or uncomfortable, observe these feelings with detachment, and, when your mind quiets, return to your focus.

Continue your focus on rising-falling. When you experience moments of emptiness, remain in that state, carefully observing the purity, spaciousness, and serenity of presence without mind-talk. During such moments spontaneous insights may emerge. Note them, and then return to your focus on the breath. When you sense that thirty minutes have passed, glance at your watch. If time is left, return to the process until the full time has elapsed. When finished, open your eyes and remain quiet in your chair for several minutes, reorienting yourself to the room.

Each time you practice, your experience of the exercise may change. This is to be expected and not to be judged. There are no right or wrong experiences, just differences.

QUICK RECAP OF MINDFULNESS TRAINING EXERCISE

- Sit in a quiet place with eyes closed, feet uncrossed, and hands resting comfortably on your thighs.
- Begin with a deep breath and then return to your normal breathing pattern, counting each cycle of inhalation and exhalation. Count

ten cycles. If you lose count begin again. When completed count two more sequences of ten breaths each.

- After counting a total of thirty breaths, focus on the rising and falling of your abdomen that naturally occurs with each inhalation and exhalation of the breath.
- Anchor your attention on the breath. When distracted, observe what the mind is doing and then return to your focus.
- If you experience moments when your mind is empty and completely still, experience this state, and then return to your breathing focus.
- During the course of this exercise, if your mind is overly active use Exercise 4: a Modified Mindfulness Training.

It is very important to practice mindfulness on a daily basis both as a structured training exercise, and in daily activities. If you cannot work it in to your morning schedule try it on the bus to work, during lunch hour, a break, or in the evening. If thirty minutes is difficult, start with fifteen. Do not blame yourself if you have not kept it up regularly (this is more mind-talk), just begin again. Each time it will be different. There are no good sessions or bad sessions. Just follow the exercise and accept the experience as it occurs.

Some individuals already have a daily meditation in the form of prayer or a specific technique. Mindfulness training is likely somewhat different as it teaches the skill of careful observation. It is important to remember that mindfulness training is not about pleasure or bliss, it is about being awake to the present moment and discovering the truth of one's life. If your meditation time is exclusively spent in the peace of relaxation, and you are delightfully lost in the pleasure, your mind will have again taken you over and left you unaware of the present moment. Without an effort at careful observation and mindfulness, you will lose the opportunities mindfulness training can offer.

EXERCISE 4:

A MODIFIED MINDFULNESS TRAINING EXERCISE (FOR INDIVIDUALS WITH A RESTLESS MIND)

To counteract a very active mind, focus on the activity of your mind. Give your mind a large field to play in. Observe it, the thoughts, feelings, images, and sensations that enter and leave without becoming absorbed in the mind-talk. Do this the way a journalist would observe a news event. Become a reporter on the activities of your mind. Observe the character of your mind-talk. Identify thoughts, images, feelings, and sensations. Are they past or current? At what speed does your mind move? Keep observing your mind. Do not get involved with it. In time, your mind will slow down and quiet itself. When it has done so, refocus on your breathing and resume Exercise 3.

This approach to mindfulness training is very helpful when the mind is very active. This can be further supplemented by controlled breathing Exercises 7 and 10. As you work with these exercises, you will discover what works best for you. This may vary according to your level of training or the degree to which your mind is active. Feel free to explore.

EXERCISE 5:

MINDFULNESS (IN DAILY LIVING)

Read this exercise prior to a meal. Record it on an audiotape allowing thirty minutes. At the conclusion of the tape you will have an additional thirty or more minutes to complete your meal. *

Place the prepared food and all that is necessary for your meal in front of you. Remain quietly in your chair for five minutes. Allow your mind and body to become still, leave the matters of the day, and center on the eating process. The meal is to be taken in silence over a period of one hour with slow and deliberate movements.

Begin by observing the food in front of you. Notice its shape, texture, color, and aroma. Notice how the utensils and foods play against each other. Notice the warmth or coolness of the food. Slowly choose how you will begin the meal, and then raise the utensil.

---

* This exercise is a modified version of an exercise presented at a workshop by Ram Dass.

Place the food in your mouth and notice its texture against your body, its temperature, and its touch. Slowly chew your food, drawing your attention to all the sensations. Take as long as possible to chew the food as you experience the mechanical aspects of digestion; the movement of the jaw, teeth, and tongue, the salivary juices, the slow breakdown of the food, and the change in texture and taste. When ready, swallow the food, observing its movement into your esophagus and stomach. Pause to allow the food to digest. (pause five minutes)

You are now ready for your next forkful of food. As you chew this forkful, become aware of the deeper essence of the food. It incorporates the elements of the earth, the nurturing of the farmer, and the preparation in your home, all so you may live. It is life giving to life. (pause five minutes)

You are now ready for your third forkful. Become aware of how eating is the symbol of sacrifice. The sky sacrificed rain for the food to grow, the earth sacrificed its nutrients, the plant its fruit. In turn, we sacrifice as we serve life. (pause five minutes)

Food is the life of all beings; and all food comes from the rain above. Sacrifice brings the rain from heaven, and sacrifice is sacred action.

"Sacred action . . . comes from the Eternal, and therefore is the Eternal ever present in a sacrifice." (*The Bhagavad Gita*)

Take your next forkful of food. Become aware of how this food, a product of the sky and the earth will become part of the chemicals and structural elements of your mind and body. This food represents your union with all that is, and all that will be. (pause five minutes) Notice how filled you can become without a large quantity of food.

With your next forkful, experience the grace of life giving to life.

"We don't say grace *before* meals. We say it *with* meals. Or rather we don't *say* grace; we *chew* it.

"Grace is the first mouthful of each course—chewed and chewed until there is nothing left of it. And all the time you're chewing you pay attention to the flavor of the food, to its consistency and temperature, to the pressures on your teeth and the feel of the muscles in your jaws.

". . . . attention to the experience of something given,
something you haven't invented, not the memory of a form of
words addressed to someone in your imagination." (*Island*,
Aldous Huxley)

Return to the meal and continue as you have begun. Slowly,
with reverence, complete your ingestion of the food (using a
total of one hour from the beginning of this exercise), at all
times being mindful of the experience. When you have finished
remain in silence for an additional five minutes, aware at all
times of the present moment.

Following the exercise, observe what you have learned. The first thing
I usually hear is "I can't believe how filled I feel." When doing this exercise at the workshop we usually go immediately to a silent lunch. After
lunch I usually hear "I ate very little; I was not even hungry." This was a
particularly important revelation for an individual that came to a workshop seeking a way to deal with a persistent weight problem. My observation is that our sense of hunger is directly related to our level of relaxation,
the quietness of our mind, mindful eating, and the pace of eating. You
can make a note of your own observations, and consider the value and
importance of silence, sacredness, and mindfulness as a part of eating.

CONCLUSION

Learning and practicing mindfulness is not easy, and, perhaps, not for
everyone. It is important to continue your practice of mindfulness, both
in your daily activities and the thirty-minute daily practice session.
Those whose minds are difficult to quiet will find mindfulness training
easier after physical exercise, at a quiet time of the day, as part of a
regular mindfulness training group, or in the context of a life-style that
gives priority to quiet time alone. The few who continue to find mindfulness difficult may wish to consider structured relaxation programs such
as biofeedback, progressive relaxation, or guided imagery (see chapter 6). Mastering these approaches makes mindfulness training easier.

Now that we have explored the basics of the first component of
healing, mindfulness, we are ready to learn more about healing and its
second component, self-regulation.

Chapter 4

SELF-REGULATION

IN THE PRECEDING chapter we learned about mindfulness, and, in this chapter, we will learn about the second component of healing: self-regulation. Together, these natural, powerful, and uniquely human capacities enable us to assume a remarkable level of control over our mind and body.

We are accustomed to regulating and changing our external environment. If it is cold, we put more clothes on or turn up the thermostat. If we are allergic to cats, we avoid them. We do not devote special attention to these changes—we make them quickly and easily. In self-healing, the goal is to use our power to make changes in a different way. Instead of manipulating the outside world, we shift our focus to regulating and controlling the inner environment of our mind and body: attitude, thoughts, emotions, feelings, biochemistry, and physiology. Working with our inner environment allows us to choose consciously how our mind and body will work.

The idea of the body as a self-regulating system is not new. In 1932, the Harvard physiologist, Walter B. Cannon, formulated the concept of homeostasis to describe the tendency of the mind and body to maintain its balance.

Just as a building has a thermostat that regulates its heat or air conditioning, we each have a built-in mechanism that automatically regulates the various functions of our body. Examples of homeostasis are numerous. The body has mechanisms for turning on and off the production of hormones, balancing the clotting and bleeding factors, regulating blood pressure, pulse, and respiration, and the acidity and alkalinity of the body fluids. Within certain limits, homeostasis keeps our mind and body healthy. Because our mind and body work as a single system, any excessive stress or strain leads to imbalance. We call this disease.

Cannon believed that regulation of the body occurs automatically and is not subject to conscious control. This automaticity occurs through the body's ability to sense an imbalance and then direct a corresponding change to restore balance, like the feedback loop of a furnace and thermostat in a heating system. The thermostat's capacity to register temperature maintains a mechanical mindfulness of the system. When the thermostat measures a deviation from the set temperatures, it regulates the system by turning the furnace on or off.

Cannon's work was preceded by related research that specifically focused on the human capacity for self-regulation. In the early 1900s, Johannes H. Schultz, a German psychiatrist and neurologist interested in the reported self-regulatory achievements of Indian yogis, began to study and test this capacity in ordinary individuals.[1] His important research suggested that homeostasis, regulation of the mind-body system, may in fact not be fully automatic but subject to voluntary, conscious control. By teaching individuals in regular training sessions to repeat a simple directive statement to their bodies, "My right hand is warm, my right hand is warm," Schultz discovered that, within a period of time, individuals could, in fact, warm their hands. His trainees had intervened to self-regulate the circulatory system, a system previously thought to be automatic. Eventually, Schultz developed a series of exercises that trained individuals to voluntarily 1) relax the muscular system, 2) control the vascular system, 3) regulate the heart rate, and 4) enhance the respiratory system.

In the late 1960s and early 1970s, Dr. Elmer Green and his wife Alyce Green of the Menninger Clinic, assisted by other researchers, extended Schultz's work and developed the basic process of biofeedback, which is machine-assisted self-regulation. Biofeedback assists the untrained individual to detect subtle physiologic changes in the body.

Through an electrical monitoring device, the machinery records electrical impulses from selected muscles, skin temperature, or a variety of other easily measured mind-body functions and feeds these signals back to the person in the form of tones or visual displays. The individual thus has electronically enhanced information about his or her internal condition. This monitoring and reporting of one's biology is called biofeedback. When a user wishes to create a specific change in muscle tension or skin temperature, he or she can in time learn how to accomplish this change by creating certain inner body feelings or images which, through mind-body linkages, achieve the desired result.

Figure 4.1 illustrates how a self-regulatory systems works. Whether through 1) the natural process of homeostasis, or 2) machine-assisted biofeedback, such a system requires a sensing device that "senses and knows" the status of the system and a regulatory device that initiates action to adjust the system.

Biofeedback uses easily measurable biologic information, muscle tension, and skin temperature, to assist individuals in learning self-regulation. But what about the more subtle biochemical and physiologic aspects of the mind-body that we would also like to self-regulate?

In the 1970s Dr. Herbert Benson, a research physician at Harvard medical school, began working with individuals who were learning and practicing a technique of meditation called Transcendental Meditation (commonly called TM). He was able to demonstrate that this technique can regulate heart rate, blood pressure, the amount of oxygen that is used by the body for metabolism, and a variety of other physiologic functions. Expanding on his research, others have demonstrated

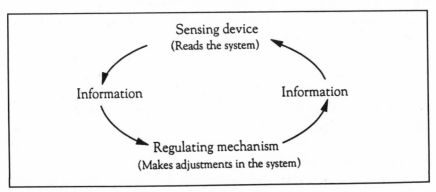

Figure 4-1. A self-regulating system.

that this technique can regulate brain waves, heart rhythms, the muscular activity of the gastrointestinal system, and, as discussed in chapter 2, the immune and hormonal systems.

It now appears that most aspects of the mind and body can be controlled, to some extent, through conscious effort. All that is needed is a finely tuned sensing device (for humans, this is mindfulness) to tell us what is going on and the skills and will to activate our self-regulatory capacities.

THE TWO COMPONENTS OF SELF-REGULATION

Self-regulation has two components, conscious living and daily practices. In contrast to living on automatic pilot, conscious living is choosing to think and act in healthy ways. It is being awake rather than asleep, proactive rather than reactive. Examples of conscious living (to be discussed in more detail in chapters 5, 6, and 7) include the choice of healthy attitudes such as honesty, simplicity, and contentment, and the integration into daily life of the life-styles that flow from these attitudes.

Conscious living trains the mind by relying on its natural propensity to create habits. When we are engrossed in unhealthy habits, we fail to recognize and use effectively this natural tendency. Instead, we hopelessly persist in unhealthy and unsatisfying behavior. By practicing healthy attitudes and behaviors, even when our minds, unconvinced of their value, continue to be drawn to the momentary pleasure of unhealthy ones, we will slowly and permanently establish new, healthier, and more pleasurable habits.

In addition to creating new and healthier habits, conscious living helps to regulate the mind in three additional ways: 1) it suppresses the emergence of their opposites (for example, truthfulness suppresses and eventually eradicates the tendency to lie), 2) it promotes good will and harmony with others and with the environment (in this manner it reduces mental conflict and mind-talk), and 3) it further trains the mind in mindfulness.

Acting as if our minds were already naturally compelling us toward healthy attitudes and life-styles takes both effort, constant attention, the support of others, and, most importantly, because conscious living is an action, it requires intention and will. It is not easy. It requires 1) thinking and acting in opposition to mind-styles and life-styles that have been present for many years, 2) letting go of things, that although comfortable and familiar, do not work, and 3) beginning to think and act in ways that differ from family and societal norms. Unfortunately, it often takes a major disruption to our lives; illness, loss of a loved one, uncontrollable anxiety, or the persistent fatigue and distress that comes with unending dissatisfaction with life, to awaken us to new possibilities and provide the intention and will necessary for conscious living. It is too often true that we must first become ill before we can summon forth sufficient awareness and intention to become well.

The second aspect of self-regulation is daily practices. Daily practices are specific activities such as mindfulness training, breath control, aerobic conditioning, biofeedback, and nutritional practices that are directed towards regulating specific aspects of the mind and body. Because any new practice requires time, effort, and focus, it is important to be precise in choosing one that is right for you.

In my medical practice and personal life, I learned the importance of carefully evaluating each phase of life to determine which self-regulatory practices would be both appropriate and timely. I start by examining what is happening in the present moment in the individual's life. Is there a problem with stress, headaches, colitis, fatigue, anxiety, or another physical or emotional disorder? If an individual is feeling anxious or sick, this *must* be dealt with first. As the overt symptoms of distress resolve, the focus can then shift to further healing and health promotion.

Daily practices must be learned, scheduled into the day, and practiced with effort and persistence. Working with a new practice, it is important to evaluate its effect continually, and, if necessary, fine-tune it until we meet with success. Eventually, it will become a new habit—as we recognize and appreciate the delight that comes from taking charge of our minds and bodies, we will gravitate toward this new habit, thereby diminishing the need for further forced effort. It is not necessary to begin with a major new practice. At times small changes may be the best way to begin (see Fifty Ways to Begin, chapter 9). What is important is that we do what we can and do it with full attention.

ASPECTS OF SELF-REGULATION

As we explore the dynamics of self-regulation, it is important to understand some of its important aspects: These include 1) appropriateness, 2) timeliness, and 3) measurability.

To be effective, self-regulation must respond appropriately to our life situation with changes that result in mental and physiologic balance and well-being. We have the capacity to direct our minds in healthy or unhealthy ways. An example of this can be seen in an individual's reaction to stress. Of the available options in coping with stress (denial, avoidance, withdrawal, submissive compliance, medication, or self-understanding through mindfulness) the last of these options is rarely chosen, although it is, at all times, the most appropriate. Although temporary action (treatment) to reduce stress, may be an appropriate first step toward lessening or reducing feelings of anxiety, it is inappropriate for the long-term goal of full health. Mindfulness, a more appropriate long-term strategy, in combination with self-regulation, permanently shifts and changes our emotional and physical reaction to stress.

To know which changes are appropriate, we must rely on our body feeling. Do we feel healthier? Do we feel a state of well-being? Ultimately, we must determine, by ourselves, what is appropriate for our lives, turning, when helpful, to written information and advice from those we trust.

Self-regulatory changes must also be timely. Again, stress is a good example. Individuals suffering from stress initially try many inappropriate responses to stress, such as denial or avoidance. Then, they endure the physical and emotional consequence of stress: overt anxiety, headaches, high blood pressure, stomach distress, or disturbed interpersonal relationships. Then, finally, out of desperation they seek appropriate guidance in self-regulation. The latter consequences of stress often require treatment that assists in reducing the immediate symptoms but does not lead to healing. Only after relieving the severe symptoms can we begin what would have been helpful much earlier: mindfulness and timely self-regulation. The time to deal with imbalance is *early* not late.

Other problems, when responded to in a delayed and untimely manner, are considerably more costly to both the individual and the culture. Heart disease, the number-one killer and source of disability in the United States, is such an example. Today, we are aware of most of the major risk factors for heart disease: hypertension, smoking, poor nutrition, lack of exercise, and an overreactive, compulsive, stress-inducing personality—behaviors often present many years before the onset of overt disease. As a physician, I see the end products of inappropriate and untimely responses to each of these unhealthy habits. Finally, at middle age, after the crises of broken hearts or the confrontations with death, many are ready for healthy change. The untimeliness of this response costs society in dollars and individuals in the quality and longevity of life.

A final comment on timeliness. It is always distressing to speak with individuals who discover late in life that, although they have done everything "right," they have deferred and deferred joy and peace until there is no time left. When I ask individuals in my workshops what percentage of their time is peaceful or joyful, the answer is invariably very little. Ask yourself that question. Timely self-regulation results in adding years of quality to one's life.

In addition to appropriateness and timeliness, self-regulatory change needs to be measurable. We can measure change in the mind-body system by observing our state of well-being (level of feelings of wellness, wholeness, calmness, confidence, competence, etc.), or in our physiology (lowered blood pressure, diminished headaches, decreased muscle tension, enhancement of our immune system, reduction in the activity of the autonomic nervous system, etc.)

Each of these measurements is a form of biofeedback. They tells us how far we have shifted the workings of our mind-body from adapting improperly and causing disease, to promoting health. Even though we cannot measure health and wholeness with instruments, with mindfulness and self-regulation, we become increasingly familiar with the inner experience of well-being. Using this as an inner marker, we develop an increasing ability to assess and self-direct our lives towards health.

APPLYING SELF-REGULATION

Self-regulation is a much different process than mindfulness. Whereas mindfulness is the capacity to precisely observe our present moment inner and outer experience, self-regulation is the capacity to act and change our experience. Both are essential.

Unlike the treatment model, self-regulatory actions are self-directed, rely on our inner resources, and are, at all times, directed not at fixing what is wrong, but at the expansion and enhancement of our lives. Using this new approach, you will discover that chapters 5, 6, and 7, which examine the applications of self-regulation, are organized to reflect the use of the two components of the healing process, mindfulness and self-regulation. When reading these chapters, first decide what you want in your life, not what you want to get rid of. This may be a new experience.

The three major applications of self-regulation are as follows:

General relaxation
Regulation of the body
Regulation of the mind

GENERAL RELAXATION

For most individuals, daily life is very stressful. Much of the illness seen in a typical doctor's office is either directly or indirectly related to personal or job stress. As a result, learning to relax the mind and body (the topic of chapter 5) is usually the first attempt at self-regulation.

There are many approaches to general relaxation. They include mindfulness training, biofeedback, exercise, yoga, healthy nutritional practices, controlled breathing, imagery, and the many activities we can each draw upon from our personal experience such as quietly reading, going for a walk, or taking time for ourselves. The specific effects of each technique may vary as may the situation in which each is most effective. The following two reports demonstrate how general relaxation practices are currently being evaluated in medical research.

Dr. Chandra Patel and his colleagues, reporting in *British Medical Journal*, documented the effects of general relaxation in reducing the risks of disease and promoting health.[2] They gave health education advice accompanied by training in breathing exercises and meditation to a group of individuals who were at high risk for coronary heart disease. A control group of similar individuals continued their usual sources of medical care. At the end of four years, the group using relaxation practices had a lower incidence of heart disease, fewer fatal heart attacks, and less evidence of coronary insufficiency.

Dr. Dean Ornish, reporting in the British medical journal *Lancet*, studied the use of general relaxation techniques in a group of patients suffering from coronary heart disease.[3] These patients received three weeks of intensive relaxation training, and a healthy, low salt, vegetarian diet. The relaxation practices included stretching/relaxation exercises, meditation, and visualization. When compared to a controlled group of similar individuals, they achieved a 44 percent increase in their exercise capacity, improved function of the -heart, a 20.5 percent decrease in cholesterol, and a 91 percent reduction in anginal episodes.

As you will notice in these reports, it is not unusual for medical researchers to focus on the objective and measurable results of their experiments, leaving to our imagination any healing or health promoting effects that are not as easily measurable and so are considered soft data.

REGULATING THE BODY

The second application of self-regulation is in regulating the body. Although there is much we know, we are still in the very early stages of learning how to self-regulate many of the systems in our body. In chapter 6, we will review four major body systems (cardiovascular, respiratory, gastrointestinal, and immune) and explore the practices that are currently available to self-regulate each of these systems. The following two research reports are examples of current research in this area.

Evaluating the role of physical fitness in self-regulating the body Dr. Steven Blair and his colleagues, writing in JAMA, reported on a study in which they tested the fitness levels of thirteen thousand men and woman over an eight-year period.[4] There was a striking decrease in death from all causes, including cardiovascular disease and cancer in those individuals, men and woman, who were physically fit. It is likely that this decrease in mortality was directly related to the metabolic and cardiorespiratory effects of exercise, which include conditioning the heart, lowering the pulse rate, decreasing the risk of high blood pressure, and enhancing the immune system.

Writing in the same journal, Dr. Walter M. Bortz reported on his observations that many of the metabolic and functional changes in the body that are commonly attributed to the aging process (these changes occur in almost all of the body's systems) are quite similar to changes observed subsequent to a period of forced physical inactivity. He raises the intriguing question: Are these changes caused by aging or a lifetime of inactivity that deconditions the body? His opinion is that exercise may be a simple, yet extraordinary practice for regulating the body.

REGULATING THE MIND

Applying self-regulation to the mind is the single most important self-healing skill. The mind can create a life of wholeness and health, or disease and suffering. The former is our birthright and can be seen most clearly in young children whose sense of wonder, confidence, trust, resilience, curiosity, connectedness, and wholeness has not as yet been eroded by the unhealthy teachings of immature parents and teachers or the forced adherence to unhealthy social and cultural value systems. The disease and suffering results from imposition and programming of these unhealthy and impersonal perspectives on to the natural gifts of a child.

Regulating the mind, reclaiming our birthright and adult right to self-determine and self-choose the content of our minds, is essential for full health. For this, we are compelled to become mindful of our lives, treat them seriously, and bring to them the consciousness and practices that will enable us to move beyond the repetitive unhealthy pro-grammed patterns that determine our lives to a truthful and compre-hensive understanding of who and what we are: an understanding that will free us to live and choose what is right and appropriate in each moment of our lives. Without this commitment, life continues to be lived automatically through the conditioning of past experience recol-lected as mind-talk, and we forever lose contact with our capacity for mindfulness and the healthy tendencies that are natural to the un-tainted child. There are no other options, either we run the mind, or it runs us.

The mind's power stems from its capacity, when trained, to precisely observe and direct itself and the body. This natural ability of the brain, often underutilized and poorly understood by science (even when one considers the magnificent discoveries and contributions of PNI research), has been a source of inspiration and study for millennia. This last category of self-regulation will be further explored in chapter 7.

Components	Conscious living
	Daily pratices
Aspects	Appropriate
	Timely
	Measurable
Applications	General relaxation
	Regulation of the body
	Regulation of the mind

Figure 4.2. Self-regulation.

THE LIMITS OF SELF-REGULATION

As new concepts of mind and body have emerged, some of us have come to infer that all physical disease is caused by unhealthy attitudes, and that the mind can control all aspects of the body. Others have suggested the opposite, that physical health will result in mental health, and the body controls the mind. These are both commonly held beliefs. We might call the former "new age thinking" and the latter "traditional medical thinking."

Anyone who has experienced mental stress can testify that the mind has a major effect on the body. Similarly, anyone who has cared for an individual with Alzheimer's disease or with the intractable pain of cancer can be quickly convinced of the enormous power of the body to shrink consciousness. There can be little question of the interactiveness of mind and body; at times they work together and at times one can overwhelm the other.

Severe emotional disease can occur in the most fit of bodies, and severe physical disease can occur with the most fit of minds. Dyslexia, Alzheimer's disease, and schizophrenia are examples of disorders that afflict the brain that are minimally, if at all, subject to self-regulation. The same can be said of predominantly physical disorders such as sickle cell anemia, Huntington's Chorea, and many other genetic disorders.

These are largely unrelated to attitudes or life-styles. We can, through our physical and mental responses to these disorders, shape their impact on our lives, but we cannot change the reality of their existence.

It is untrue, unfair, and inappropriate, in the excitement of the discovery of our capacity for mindfulness and self-regulation, to ignore the reality that our body and mind are part of the natural order of life. We cannot permanently stop the physical changes of aging or the physical death of our body. We cannot contain all the disorders that can afflict our mind and body. Nor can we become attached to the belief that we can fully create our physical and mental reality.

There is much, however, that we can control. We *can* control and move beyond worry, fear and their result, mental and physical suffering. We *can* prevent the onset of many of the diseases that impair our health; and by using our capacity for mindfulness and self-regulation, it is possible to expand and deepen our lives, discovering the possibility of living with peace, harmony, and joy.

What separates us from the plants and animals is our ability to be mindful and aware of our lives and through mindfulness self-regulate and self-determine our present and future. This uniquely human capacity provides each of us with our only opportunity for physical, mental, and spiritual freedom. Anything less than full cultivation of these two approaches to life deprives us of freedom and the capacity to realize fully our nature and its possibilities.

Chapters 5, 6, and 7 will assist you in further developing your mindfulness and self-regulatory skills. These chapters will expand upon the three ways of applying self-regulation: general relaxation, regulation of the body, and regulation of the mind.

Chapter 5

ACHIEVING
GENERAL RELAXATION

THE PRECEDING CHAPTER described self-regulation, and its three applications, general relaxation, regulation of the body, and regulation of the mind. In this and the following two chapters, we will learn how to use self-regulation to 1) quiet the mind and body, 2) restore and maintain optimal physiologic function, and 3) establish healthy and life enhancing attitudes. Because stress is so common in our daily lives, we will begin by working with the first of these three, general relaxation.

Stress is not a modern phenomena. In an Oriental culture three thousand years ago, men and women subject to the human condition, like ourselves, observed as we have that distress is inseparable from the human experience. In an attempt to understand the problems of living, and to develop ways to relieve pain and suffering, they looked inward. Some of these people devoted their entire lives to inner reflection, often in quiet meditation. They concluded from their research that troubled thinking leads to distress and disease, and they designed an approach for moving beyond suffering to full health. The approach was called yoga.

Yoga, as we know it now, is a system for healing and wholeness that uses meditation, special breathing techniques called Pranayama, and a series of physical postures called Asanas, to help individuals attain a clear understanding of their lives and their capacities to self-regulate mind and body. The founders of yoga fostered the idea that clear thinking, proper attitude, and a healthy life-style made the relief of pain, suffering, and disease a possibility in each human life. They recognized the essential truth that stress was a result of inner circumstances rather than outer circumstances.

Centuries later, in our own culture, two contemporary researchers, Thomas H. Holmes and Richard H. Rahe, in their search to understand the sources of human distress and illness, asked a similar question from a slightly different perspective. "What factor," they asked, "is common in the lives of individuals that succumb to disease?" They discovered that illness frequently occurs six to eighteen months following a cluster of stressful life events usually associated with anxiety and suffering. They observed that stress, mental and physiologic distress, was, for many individuals, the common source of acute and chronic disease.[1]

Others soon began to ask, "Why, given the same stressful situation (for example, loss of a job), do different individuals respond with differing levels of stress?" What one individual considered to be stressful, another considered a healthy challenge. Some of us appeared to be hardier and more resistant to stress; others appeared to be resigned to it.

Suzanne Kobassa, doing research at the University of Chicago, studied "hardiness," the personal qualities that convey resistance to stress-induced illness.[2] She compared two groups of middle- and upper-level executives exposed to equivalent amounts of stress. One group suffered from stress without getting ill. Individuals in the other group became ill. The former group showed more "hardiness"; a stronger commitment to self, an attitude of vigorousness toward the environment, a sense of meaningfulness, and inner feelings of confidence and competence.

Like the yogis, we are coming to understand that individuals, their attitudes, perspectives, and life-styles were central in determining responses to outside events, and thus central to the presence or absence of stress and disease. Contemporary research has led back to the mind and its role in stress.

THE WORKINGS OF THE MIND REVISITED

What is the role of the mind in stress? Simply put, unhealthy psycho-logic information causes stress. In chapter 3 we discussed the two activities of the mind—mind-talk and mindfulness. We defined mind-talk as the conscious recollection of stored information from earlier life experiences and categorized the information as factual and psychologic. We learned in chapter 3 (see Figure 3-3), that psychologic information can be both healthy and unhealthy. Mind-talk that results from stored unhealthy psychologic information is often the predominant activity of the mind and the source of stress.

Also, we saw in chapter 3 that unhealthy mind-talk reflected in troubling thoughts, images, sensations, and feelings draws our attention to its inner dialogue. Consider a thought about work or a relationship that occupies your mind day and night. You cannot move from it. It becomes an obsession. At such times you are not only absorbed in the thought but possessed by it because you have no control over it. You are in effect living a series of intense dramas around which your life is often organized.

These inner dramas have little relationship to the actual events of daily life. They establish their own momentum and rarely, if ever, assist you in resolving the dilemma at hand. In actuality, these dramas bring us back to the unresolved and often unremembered childhood wound-ings and the protective and defensive responses that we learned to use as children in order to survive the painful moments. The replay of old unhealthy psychologic mind-talk rather than the specific outer circum-stances of life, is usually the underlying source of worry, fear, and stress. We cannot permanently move beyond stress until we reduce and elimi-nate the impact of unhealthy psychologic mind-talk.

It is important to remember that the mind does not live in isolation. As recognized by the yogis and the researchers in PNI, the mind is a component of the larger system, our human organism. As such, its thoughts, images, sensations, and feelings are transformed by the brain into chemicals and nerve impulses that act as messengers passing infor-mation back and forth between the mind and body (as discussed in chapter 2). These chemical messengers cause a shift in the physiology of our body, altering it to conform to the movements of our mind. It is increasingly clear that our mental attitudes result in specific biochemical patterns in our bodies. When we become absorbed in the inner dramas of unhealthy mind-talk the result is mental and physiologic distress and imbalance.

Current research is affirming and further defining the uniqueness of each individual's response to "stressors." For example, studying chronic pain syndromes, which are a source of continuous stress [in this case temperomandibular joint (TMJ) pain], Joseph Marbach and his associates discovered that, considered as a group, no differences in immune functions were seen in individuals suffering from TMJ syndrome when compared to a healthy control group. There was, however, a suppression of certain aspects of the immune response in specific individuals suffering from "demoralization." Demoralization appears to be related to feelings of helplessness, powerlessness, and hopelessness. These latter mental attitudes are uniquely present in an individuals life *only* when early life experiences taught helplessness and powerlessness in contrast to confidence and competence. This and other related research further confirm how each of our minds and bodies react to stress differently according to our early life experiences and adult mind-talk. Figure 5.1 summarizes the chain of events that begins with unhealthy mind-talk and leads to illness.

Hans Selye, the Canadian physiologist who first detailed the physiology of stress has carefully observed the body's reaction to fear, anxiety, and emotional distress. The body's response, he noted, was a survival mechanism for our primitive ancestors, who frequently confronted real physical danger. A strong response in the face of danger activated their bodies and prepared them for coping with imminent attack—the "fight-or-flight" response. Unlike our primitive ancestors, we no longer encounter lions in the bush, instead, we create them in our heads. The "lions in our head," the daily worries of modern life, keep our minds in a state of fear, worry, and anxiety and our bodies in a state of activation and physiologic stress. Unlike the real lions, who either attack or run, they are with us for extended periods of time.[3]

What is the outcome of this constant state? The activated body responding to mental distress is entirely different from the body at rest. The pulse elevates, breathing is erratic, blood pressure increases, muscles are tense, blood is shifted from the skin and less critical areas of the body to the essential internal organs, hormone levels elevate, and the immune system is suppressed. Over the short term, these changes can

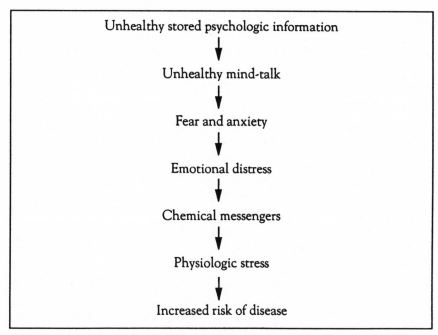

Figure 5-1. The stress response.

worsen an existing disease and/or produce a variety of new symptoms such as headaches, stomach ulcers or distress, skin conditions, suscep-tibility to infections, fatigue, and insomnia.

Selye believed that, over long periods of time, stress depletes the body of available energy and accelerates natural aging and deterioration of the body. Our current understanding of the diseases of premature aging and deterioration (among which are heart disease, cancer, high blood pressure, and musculoskeletal degeneration) is consistent with Selye's viewpoint that persistent unrelenting stress ages the body by signifi-cantly distorting its normal physiologic balance.

The research in PNI, building upon the work of Selye and others, has specifically focused on the effect of stress on the function of the immune system. Steroids and other neuropeptide transmitters, released by the brain at times of stress, appear to reduce immune surveillance, which is our natural defense against infectious agents and abnormal (cancerous) cells. This, and other observations in current neuroscientific research, increasingly support the relationship between stress, immune dysfunc-tion, and disease. This is the modern day equivalent of the conclusion reached intuitively by the ancient yogis three thousand years ago.

HEALING STRESS THROUGH MINDFULNESS AND SELF-REGULATION

Our increasing knowledge about stress is reflected, in part, in current stress-management literature, which is voluminous. Among the many approaches are time management, assertiveness, communication training, goal setting, cognitive restructuring, etc. Each of these is a valuable skill in "managing" stress. But none of these offers the possibility of *eliminating* unnecessary stress by addressing it at its source, unhealthy and inaccurate psychologic mind-talk.

How then do we begin to deal at the source? Earlier we indicated that a program for self-healing must focus on the two components of healing: mindfulness and self-regulation. The first component, mindfulness, approaches stress through the mind. It 1) helps us to experience a quiet mind, for some individuals for the first time, 2) allows us to watch our mind and learn how it works to create stress, 3) assists us in observing and working with our unhealthy psychologic mind-talk, and 4) provides us with an awareness of our mind-body that enables us to initiate self-regulatory actions.

The second component, self-regulation, approaches stress through the body by 1) relaxing the muscles, 2) controlling breathing, 3) activating relaxation-inducing neuropeptides through aerobic exercise, 4) activating the parasympathetic nervous system through the use of biofeedback and guided imagery, an action that can "deaccelerate" the mind and body, 5) reducing the intake of stimulants such as caffeine and refined sugar, and 6) living consciously through attitudes and actions that directly result in a less stressful life (see chapter 7). The body can be used to quiet the mind, which, in turn, results in a further quieting of the body. Quiet mind—quiet body. Quiet body—quiet mind.

It is unnecessary and ineffective to practice all of these mind-body techniques. It is better to master one or two and use them regularly. The mindfulness training exercise is an essential first step. It should be practiced thirty minutes each day. This can be supplemented with one of the practices listed above that focuses on the body. With this program you will notice within the first few days an increased control over your mind and body reflected in a calmer and less reactive approach to daily life.

It likely will be necessary for you to go further to discover and identify through self-observation, concentration (see chapter 7), and, if necessary, counseling, the "wounded child" within you. Two good resources for information and exercises that will help you discover your "wounded child" are John Bradshaw's books *The Family* and *Homecoming*. With continued practice and patience and insight, stress will become less and less a factor in your life. It will be replaced by the harmony and peace of mindfulness and the pleasure of a relaxed body.

The exercises that follow will assist you in learning the self-regulatory practices associated with general relaxation. The mindfulness training exercise is not repeated here, it can be found in chapter 3 as Exercise 3. Using mindfulness to work with unhealthy psychologic mind-talk will be the topic of chapter 7.

EXERCISE 6:

TENSE-RELAX

The following exercise will 1) enhance your awareness of the possible range of muscle tension and relaxation and 2) promote general relaxation through relaxing the body. Record the text on an audiocassette, observing the pauses as described. Begin by lying comfortably on your back on the floor. Allow twenty-five minutes for this exercise.

Begin with the muscles of your feet. Contract them tightly and hold the contraction for twenty seconds. (pause) Quickly release the tension and feel the relaxation moving into your feet. Notice carefully the difference between tension and relaxation. (pause twenty seconds)

Now, shift to your calf muscles and repeat the same process, contract (pause twenty seconds) and release (pause twenty seconds). When releasing notice that your feet and calves may seem heavier and warmer: a sign of increasing muscular relaxation and blood circulation to the skin and muscles. (pause twenty seconds)

Continue with the contraction of your thigh muscles. Hold (pause twenty seconds) and release (pause twenty seconds). Notice how your legs feel. Become aware of the difference between tension and relaxation. Awareness of this difference will enable you to begin self-regulation in the early stages of stress. (pause twenty seconds)

Shift your attention to the genital area. Contract (pause twenty seconds) and release (pause twenty seconds). Move to your anal area, buttocks, lower back, and abdomen. Each time, continue the same pattern, contract for twenty seconds and release for twenty seconds. Remember the twenty-second intervals as they will not be repeated again. Bring your awareness to the lower part of your body. Notice the feeling of relaxation with its heaviness and warmth. (pause three minutes)

Briefly become aware of your mind. Has it quieted? Does it seem more focused and relaxed? (pause one minute)

Move to your chest. Contract the chest muscles, then quickly let go into relaxation. As you experience your body relaxing, notice how breathing slows. It has a "velvet and silky" feel. Continue breathing in this manner.

Contract your shoulders and then relax. Notice how your shoulders, which are often held tight, sink into the body. By checking on your shoulders during the day, you can quickly assess how much tension you are holding in your body. Instruct them to relax, and notice the difference.

Move to your neck, the back of your head, scalp, eyelids, face, jaw, and lips. Contract them all at once, and then relax. As you relax your face, notice how it also can be used, particularly your jaw, as an instant check of your state of tension/relaxation.

When you have completed these movements, scan your body for any areas of retained stress (common areas are the shoulders, neck, and jaw) and relax these areas by contracting and releasing the muscles. (pause one minute)

Remain quiet, feeling the relaxation in your body. Make a mental note of how it feels, and, if possible, create an image of relaxation. Give it color, shape, or texture. Remain still and enjoy the quiet for the next ten minutes. (pause ten minutes)

Notice how your mind has shifted into a more mindful state. Make a mental note of the clear and transparent feeling of mind-body relaxation. Become aware of how working with your body can relax your mind. (pause two minutes)

It is now time to return your awareness to the immediate surroundings and resume your normal activities.

Most individuals become aware of tight muscles and the presence of stress only when the muscles begin to hurt. At this late stage, it requires considerably more effort to relax them and reverse the other physical and emotional consequences of stress, which may or may not be evident at the time (too often ulcer disease, colitis, and other ailments are the "first" sign of stress). The inability to detect stress at its earliest stages denies us the ability to know when we are stressed and to do something about it sooner rather than later. With increasing mindfulness, it becomes possible to develop a finely tuned awareness of our state of tension/relaxation, and to intervene to rebalance the mind and body before the development of illness. The value of this exercise is its ability to expand your awareness of the range of tension and relaxation that is possible in your mind and body.

EXERCISE 7:

CONTROLLED BREATHING (1)

Through the ages, controlled breathing has been an important component of self-regulation. It is no less so today. It can be used alone for general relaxation, combined with the mindfulness training exercise, or practiced as a brief interlude in a hectic stressful day. You may eventually decide to use controlled breathing for all three of these uses or just one. Although scientists are beginning to study and document its effects on the mind-body, it is unnecessary for us to await the results of their studies. Enough practical knowledge is available for individuals to begin working with controlled breathing and to begin discovering directly its profound effects.

The following exercises will work with three controlled breathing techniques. It is best to practice breathing with an empty stomach, as this will allow for greater movement of your diaphragm. Record this exercise on an audiotape allowing thirty minutes. Refer to Figure 5.2 before beginning this exercise.

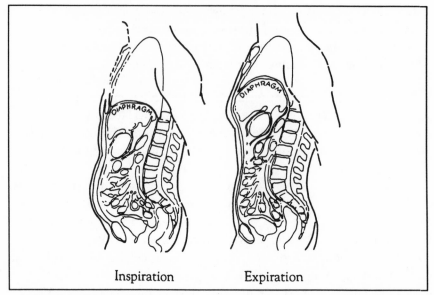

Figure 5-2. The complete breath. Reprinted from *Science of Breath*, The Himalayan Institute.

Begin by sitting on a straight backed chair or on the floor with your back against a wall. Your back should be straight, your neck elongated, and your head slightly tilted toward the ground several feet in front of you. The pressure of your body should be felt directly on the bones under your buttocks. You can check this by sliding your hands, palms up, under your buttocks until you feel the sharp protruding bones pressing on your finger tips. Your finger tips should now feel the weight of the body. Shift your body around until the maximum weight is felt. Return your hands to a resting spot on your thighs, and continue sitting in this position, which maximally expands your lungs. Close your eyes, you are ready to start the exercise.

Become aware of your breathing. Notice the depth of your exhalation and inhalation. What muscles are you using to expand and contract your chest? Most likely these are the intercostal muscles, the muscles between the ribs. Is your breathing smooth or erratic?

There are two muscles groups involved in breathing: the intercostal muscles that connect one rib to another and the diaphragmatic muscle that separates the chest cavity from the abdominal cavity. When we only use our intercostal muscles there is minimal expansion of the chest cavity; only a small amount of air can move in and out of the lungs.

Continue to observe your breathing. How much does your abdomen move when you breathe? How much movement is there from below the waist? Try to shift to abdominal and diaphragmatic breathing. We call diaphragmatic breathing a *complete breath.*

Begin by placing both your hands on your abdomen. Take a deep breath and fully exhale. Notice that the next breath will tend to come into and expand the abdomen. You will feel your hands rise. Notice the sensation. It is somewhat like blowing out the stomach and filling it like a balloon. After filling your abdomen, draw the air up through the chest by expanding the chest muscles. Move from the lower chest to the upper chest, and then to the shoulders and collar bones, drawing in the final amount of air necessary to expand the upper reaches of the lung cavity.

Exhale the air by first allowing it to flow smoothly and passively out of the chest. Then, slowly contract your abdomen until the remainder of the air in your lungs is expelled. Resume again with the inhalation sequence of abdomen, lower chest, upper chest, and collar bones and exhalation sequence of collar bones, upper chest, lower chest, and abdomen. Practice complete breathing, counting each cycle (inhalation and exhalation). Count ten breaths. If you lose count begin again at one. Count three groups of ten complete breaths each.

After counting complete breaths, begin the second component of this exercise, timed breathing. This refers to the practice of shifting the breathing cycle so that exhalation is twice the length of inhalation. Continuing with the complete breath, counting from one to four on the inhalation and from one to eight on the exhalation. The yogis suggest that on the in-breath we think of peace and relaxation, and on the out-breath we experience the entire body relaxing. You may notice that, at either the end of inhalation or exhalation, the breathing ceases for a few moments. Begin to rest your breathing at the end of expiration. This is the third aspect of the cycle: rest. If you choose to work with the rests do them with a count of one to four. They should feel effortless and should not be prolonged if you feel any discomfort or dizziness. Continue timed breathing for the next ten minutes. (pause ten minutes)

Now slow the breath down further. Decrease the volume and frequency of your breathing until you are breathing as little as possible. Notice how you can slow your mind by slowing your breathing. (pause two minutes)

You are now ready to begin the third technique: awareness of the external and internal space. The external and internal spaces of breathing may be new concepts for you. You may wish to return to this technique later for additional practice. Focus your awareness on the exhalation, and observe the distance covered by the exhaled air from the tip of the nose to the point that the breath is extended outside of your body. This is called the *external space of breathing.* You may have a sense of the distance, or you may create an image of it. You can vary it by increasing or decreasing the volume of air you expel or by varying the force of expiration. Attempt to keep the distance as small as possible by decreasing the force of the exhalation. This will, in time, diminish the exhalation. As the body quiets down, less energy is needed and less exchange of air is necessary. One of the objectives of controlled breathing is to slowly diminish the intensity of breathing until the act of breathing is soft, smooth, and almost imperceptible. Practice "feeling" the external space for five minutes. (pause five minutes)

We will now focus on the *internal space of breathing.* As the air enters the lungs, imagine it in the region of the heart. From this central point, feel it gently spreading through the body, head to foot, sensing the inner space of the body. For some, it may be helpful to image the incoming air as a white light or a gentle cleansing breeze. On exhalation, feel the air being gathered up from the body as it returns to its central point, the heart. Repeat the process again on the next inhalation. Practice this for five minutes. (pause five minutes)

Next, take ten complete breaths and then return to your normal breathing pattern. Become aware of the quietness of your breathing. Notice how smooth and regular it is. This is unlike the erratic breathing that is the normal experience for most of us. Become aware of how controlled breathing quiets the mind and body. It is a powerful self-regulatory tool. You can use it as a formal exercise or as a break in your day-to-day activities.

Open your eyes and return to the time and place of the room. Sit quietly for a few moments and notice how mindful and aware you are, how everything has slowed down, and how you can see and hear with more intensity and clarity.

Most individuals who practice breathing exercises are surprised to discover that it is possible to slow the breathing down so that it becomes almost imperceptible. The mind and body follow the breathing, relaxing in direct proportion to the slowing of the breathing process. Breathing exercises can be done for a few minutes or extended periods of time. It can be quite helpful to bring your attention to your breathing at frequent intervals during the day. This will quiet the mind and body and shift you into mindfulness.

EXERCISE 8:

GUIDED IMAGERY

Images can have a very powerful effect on the mind and body. A fearful image results in stress, a relaxing image in relaxation. Most of us respond automatically to these and other images that randomly arise in our minds or appear within our visual fields. By recognizing the power of imagery we can use it to self-direct our minds and bodies. This exercise demonstrates one way to do this.

Guided imagery uses an outside resource, usually a voice on an audiotape, to assist in the creation of a series of images that enhance relaxation. Using the text below and soft background music, you can record your own guided imagery experience. Allow thirty minutes for this exercise. Begin by lying on the floor or sitting comfortably in a chair and turning on the audiotape.

Close your eyes and take twelve complete breaths. With each in-breath you are bringing relaxation into your body, and with each out-breath you are exhaling stress. (pause one minute)

You are about to begin a journey, a journey to a very special place. It is your place, a special place you have known from the past. Perhaps it is a place you have gone for nurturing, for rest, for sorting things out. Perhaps it is a place that has brought you peace and joy. We each have a special place. For those of us who have yet to discover it, this is the time. If you cannot recall such a place, create an image of this ideal island of peace. (pause two minutes)

Take yourself back to this place. See the sights, smell the smells, hear the sounds, the touch on your skin, the air, the sun, the quiet, and the sacredness. Explore your special place and find a quiet spot to sit for a few moments. (pause two minutes)

This is a healing place. A place in which you can experience complete relaxation of your mind and body. You can feel the healing as a soft white light, or a gentle breeze cleansing and purifying, removing the stress, and reversing unhealthy habits that have accumulated over months and years. Experience your body becoming lighter, softer, warmer, and peaceful. Allow the healing to take place for the next several minutes. (pause five minutes)

It is now time to take on more energy. Bring your full awareness to the area of your heart. Experience it as full of light. Feel the light spreading to the rest of your body. With it comes warmth, vitality, a sweeping away of any residual tension, and the inward movement of calm and peace. If you wish, you may allow the light to engulf you as you, for a few moments, begin to move with the light. Enjoy this feeling and image for the next several minutes. (pause five minutes)

It is time now to return to your special place. Look around. You may discover an individual that you know can be trusted, and assist in guiding you towards the next step in your life. If you meet such a person sit with this individual and use this opportunity to ask whatever questions may be of importance to you. If you prefer to remain alone, allow yourself several minutes of meditation. It is an opportunity to reflect on important issues in your life. (pause five minutes)

This special place of yours is always available, always present for you when you wish to visit it. For a few more minutes experience it again before leaving it renewed and refreshed. (pause two minutes)

It is now time to return slowly to the time and place of the room.

Imagery is now being used by athletes, actors, musicians, artists, and others to self-regulate physiologic function, facilitate creativity, and enhance learning. The former results from the effect of images, either external images or, as in this exercise, internally created images, on the synthesis of neuropeptides (the area of the brain that generates imagery appears to be well endowed with neuropeptide-synthesizing cells), and the stimulation of other mind-body messenger systems in the brain. In this way, it is possible to create specific mental states and their physiologic equivalents through the use of imagery. This is not surprising, as we do this automatically when we are imagining fearful situations, romantic interludes, etc. The difference is in using imagery intentionally to consciously self-regulate our mind and body. For the purposes of this chapter, the emphasis has been on relaxation.

Imagery also can be used to facilitate creativity. This is one of its the most powerful uses. Imaging is invariably a process of focused attention. When the focus on an image is held, mindfulness begins and proceeds into its second stage, concentration. Mindful concentration, as previously discussed, when uncontaminated by the tendency for analytic thinking, will clear the mind and allow creative insight to emerge. With training, creativity no longer needs to be a chance event. It can be self-directed.

Finally, imagery can be used with considerable effectiveness for learning. The athlete that needs to learn a drill, the student that is learning how to spell a new word, and others who wish to practice as many times as possible before "doing," can do so in their minds. In this manner, we have the capacity to self-program our mechanical brain and teach it to work as we wish it to.

The mindfulness training exercise practiced daily, supplemented by controlled breathing, imagery, exercise, proper nutrition (modest meals low in fats, high in carbohydrates, emphasizing whole foods such as vegetables, grains, and legumes, and lacking sugar, caffeine, or preservatives), and accompanied by other practices that you have found relaxing in your life will enable you to experience relaxation on a daily basis. You will slowly recognize that your capacity to feel relaxed is not dependent on outside circumstance, but rather on your own attitudes and self-regulatory practices.

It is essential that you verify this effect through personal experience from your practice. Because it has taken time to create stress, you must be patient, it takes time to retrain the mind. The natural tendency of your mind and the natural tendency of our culture will work together to slow your efforts, so, if possible, ask a trained instructor to assist you in learning these techniques until you are comfortable with your capacity to continue alone without resistance.

As you increase your work with these stress-regulating exercises, you will begin to note increasing clarity in your life, decreased anxiety and confusion, diminished hyperactiveness, and an increased presence with yourself, work, and others. Your body, receiving new messages from the brain, will respond by returning its physiology to a normal and healthy balance.

At the beginning of this chapter, we stated that the elimination of unnecessary stress ultimately requires the reduction and elimination of unhealthy mind-talk. The knowledge gained from mindfulness training and general relaxation slowly allows the individual to recognize, first intellectually, and then emotionally, the difference between false information acquired from others and accepted as accurate and the true reality of ones deeper self that pre-exists the "acquired" information. Little more can be said. Further understanding of this statement is only possible through the perspective and experience of mindfulness.

After taking a look at regulation of the body in chapter 6, we return to the topic of unhealthy mind-talk in chapter 7, where we will explore the acquired misperceptions of powerlessness, loneliness, and deprivation.

Chapter 6

REGULATING THE BODY

IN THE PRECEDING chapter, we learned about the first category of self-regulation, general relaxation. In this chapter we will turn our attention to the body, and focus on its four major systems: the respiratory, circulatory, gastrointestinal, and immune systems. Each of these significantly affects our level of health and is responsive to conscious efforts at regulation.

We all look with awe and wonder at the agility of a ballerina, the physiologic control of a master yogi, the dexterity of an accomplished pianist, the flexibility of a gymnast, and the endurance of a long-distance runner. Such individuals, with patience, disciplined practice, and much care, have achieved extraordinary mastery over their bodies. These achievements represent examples of the capacity to attain optimal function through self-regulation of the body's systems.

In contrast, when our bodies are inadequately cared for or provided with unhealthy nutrients (impure food, air, or water), they deteriorate. Continually adjusting to unhealthy life-styles, they expend increasing amounts of energy attempting to recover their natural balance. When energy is depleted, we complain of fatigue, disturbing symptoms, and, in time, seek treatment from health professionals for serious physical distress and disease.

There is, however, a slow, yet persistent and continuous, shift in our understanding of the sources of disease and the efforts necessary for healing. This can be seen most dramatically in the ongoing search for effective strategies for the prevention and treatment of atheroclerotic heart disease (heart disease caused by deposits containing cholesterol— these deposits are found in the large and medium-sized arteries) and other diseases. In 1987, there were 976,000 deaths from coronary heart disease in our country. This represents 45.9 percent of all deaths. To counter this problem, extensive research has resulted in a continuous flow of expensive and sophisticated technologic approaches to treat-ment. Diagnostic devices and medicines that can dissolve clots and operations (coronary artery bypass and balloon angioplasty) that bypass calcium plaques and re-expand arteries are among these advances. The costs are extraordinary. One dose of the clot dissolving drug costs $1500. This year two-hundred-fifty thousand coronary bypass opera-tions will be performed costing $7 billion dollars.

The tide is turning. In 1983 (I previously referred to this research in chapter #4), in JAMA, and in 1990 in Lancet, the prestigious British medical journal, Dr. Dean Ornish presented the results of his studies on life-style interventions and their effect on the progression of heart disease. Using meditation and relaxation techniques, nutrition and exercise, he was able to clearly demonstrate an individual's capacity for reversing the abnormalities of atheroclerotic heart disease through self-regulation. Without the use of drugs or medical technology, he was able to document the reversal of atherosclerosis in the study group as com-pared to the progression of disease in the control group. These results were most marked in the groups with the greatest disease, and the results were evident in as short a period as one year.

Dr. Alexander Leaf, the noted Chief of Medicine at the Massa-chusetts General Hospital, commented on these findings in a recent editorial in the New England Journal of Medicine. He states, "It is not only the deplorable toll in lives and morbidity exacted by athero-sclerosis, however that makes the present medical response deplorable. It is also the fact that none of these interventions provide an approach that will reduce the incidence of the disease in the next generation of persons 20, 30, or 40 years old, who will be doomed to the same health consequences *unless more is done to prevent the disease.*" (italics mine) He goes further to state that "Physicians should help the public to understand that good cardiovascular health is largely an individual responsibility and there are no miraculous cures for coronary heart disease."[1]

The recognition that the human mind conveys to each of us the capacity to self-regulate our body is shifting from the domain of folklore, ancient practice, and speculation to the mainstream of modern medical science. It is becoming quite evident that the imbalances resulting from years of mental and physical neglect can, to a large extent, be prevented and reversed through individual efforts at self-healing. These efforts must not be lukewarm or tentative, but rather a thoughtful, deliberate, and persistent undertaking. Mindfulness, self-regulation, and other self-healing practices can 1) prevent the development of acute or chronic disease, 2) assist in healing disease, 3) promote optimal functioning of the mind and body, and 4) maximize our energy. In this chapter we will examine four body systems. We will first expand our understanding of how these systems work and then explore approaches to self-regulation.

THE RESPIRATORY SYSTEM

The respiratory system is a direct connection between our body and the outside world. Although we are bathed in air (as sea life is bathed in water), it is the purpose of this system to extract life-sustaining oxygen from the air and transfer it to the circulatory system for delivery to the body's cells.

It is through our nose that we first greet incoming air. The soft mucous membranes of the nose, already warmed by an extensive blood supply, in turn warm incoming air to the approximate body temperature. These membranes also extract warmth from the air traveling from the lungs to the outside environment, retrieving the warmth they provided for the inward journey. This heat exchange system assists in maintaining homeostatic balance by stabilizing the temperature inside and outside the body.

Cilia, which are small hairs, are present in the nasal cavity to remove any particulate matter in the air we inhale. These contaminants are carried away by a constantly moving stream of mucus, which is propelled by the synchronous and rhythmic movements of millions of cilia. The mucus is moved against gravity to the back of the nose and down the throat to the stomach, where it is either excreted through the bowel, or digested and returned as its chemical constituents for reuse by the body.

The warmed air passes through the upper airway, the trachea, and its branches, the bronchi, finally concluding its journey to the lung's small thin air sacs, the alveoli. These sacs are saturated with blood vessels where an exchange takes place between carbon dioxide and oxygen. Carbon dioxide, the unusable end product of human metabolism leaves the blood and passes back out the respiratory system through expiration to the air, where it will be used by the plant kingdom. The inhaled oxygen is picked up by the hemoglobin of the red blood cells, which leave the alveoli saturated with the oxygen necessary for the production of human energy. As we exhale, we return the carbon dioxide-rich air to the environment, and inhale oxygen-rich air for our needs.

Air is propelled into and out of our lungs by expansion and contraction of our chest cavity. When the breathing muscles contract, they create space in the cavity, and a vacuum is created that expands the elastic lung into the chest cavity. When the lung expands, the alveoli open, drawing in air. When the contracted muscles relax, the lungs shrink and expel air. This rhythmic cycle normally occurs twelve to sixteen times each minute.

As previously discussed, there are two phases of exhalation and inhalation. Each phase is under our voluntary control, and each affects the quantity and quality of our breathing. The first phase uses the diaphragm, a large sheet of muscle separating our chest cavity and the abdomen (Figure 5-2). When the diaphragm and abdominal muscles are actively contracted, they squeeze the lungs into the upper portion of the chest, expelling large quantities of contained air. The second phase relies on the chest muscles. When contracted, they augment the diaphragmatic muscle by expelling air from the upper lungs.

The reverse is true for inhalation. Beginning with the active contraction of the lower rib muscles, the abdominal cavity expands, creating a negative pressure that draws the diaphragm down and increases the size of the lower chest cavity resulting in an expansion of the lungs. Similarly, the contraction of the chest muscles expands the lower and then upper chest cavities.

A complete breath uses these two muscle groups. Each inhalation begins with the diaphragm, and moves to the lower and upper chest muscles. The exhalation is done in reverse. This allows for the largest expansion of the chest cavity and inhalation of oxygenated air and the most complete contraction and expulsion of deoxygenated air.

RESPIRATORY DISTRESS

Left untroubled, the intricate and well-orchestrated movement of breathing can satisfy our internal needs for many decades. Unfortunately, the air we breathe, our respiratory system, and our breathing patterns are rarely untroubled. To repeat the obvious, the air we breathe is of poor quality, which is a result of our industrial society and unhealthy habits, the most destructive of which is smoking. A brief excursion to the mountains allows us to remember the taste and smell of unpolluted air.

In addition to our exposure to cancer-inducing chemicals in cigarette smoke, smoke inhalation saturates incoming air with carbon monoxide. It is hemoglobin's job to carry oxygen, but when carbon monoxide is present, it attaches to the hemoglobin more firmly than oxygen does. Displacing oxygen, carbon monoxide reduces the quantity of oxygen that is available for the production of body energy. Cigarette smoke and other contaminants also increase the production of thick mucus and are destructive to the normal functioning of the cilia. This combined effect compromises the ability of the nasal and tracheal filtering systems to screen out unwanted pollutants, including bacteria and virus particles.

Excessive mucus falls back into the stomach and respiratory tree. In the lungs, this often infected and filthy mucus layers itself on the bronchial mucosa increasing susceptibility to bronchitis, throat irritations, chronic cough, and asthmatic symptoms. Swallowed mucus can cause an annoying sensation of nausea in the morning. Excessive mucus production can also be caused by milk products and other less well-identified food products. To some degree, we can regulate mucus production by decisions about our environment and the foods we eat.

A second major correctable source of respiratory distress, inadequate breathing, results from a lack of knowledge of proper breathing techniques, and a propensity for shallow and erratic breathing, characteristic of the breathing patterns associated with stress. As previously discussed, ancient wisdom and contemporary scientific research suggest a direct relationship between breathing patterns and states of consciousness. When we are preoccupied with mind-talk, breathing is on automatic pilot. For most of us, because mind-talk is a day-to-day pattern, this means the shallow and inadequate breathing that only uses the chest muscles, even though use of the diaphragmatic muscles is important.

When the mind is balanced and focused, breathing is full, rhythmic, and primarily uses the diaphragm. By reducing the respiratory rate, becoming mindful of the breathing process, and focusing inward, we can slow, control, and shift the mind, through control of our breathing, from mind-talk to mindfulness, relaxing both mind and body. This requires that we remain aware of our breath, and the character of our breathing, and, through self-regulation, control our breathing patterns. Our breathing pattern and our mental state are directly connected— shift one, and you automatically shift the other.

EXERCISE 9:

THE RESPIRATORY SYSTEM

This exercise, using guided imagery, will assist you in becoming more mindful of your respiratory system. Continued awareness, attention, and sensitivity to its operation and needs will enable you to initiate appropriate and timely self-regulation, for which a highly developed mindfulness is at all times a prerequisite.

Allow thirty minutes for this exercise, which should be prerecorded on an audiotape.

Find a comfortable seat or place on the ground and, seated or lying down, close your eyes. Become aware of your mental activity. Notice the mind-talk, and its movement between thoughts, images, sensations, and feelings. Draw your attention to your breathing. Are you breathing with your diaphragm, chest muscles, or both? Is there a smooth rhythm to your breathing? Is it shallow or deep? How do the rest of your muscles feel—tense or relaxed? (pause two minutes)

Bring your attention to the tip of your nose. Feel the air going into and out of your nostrils. Does it go through each nostril evenly? It probably does not. Ancient wisdom states that breathing asymmetrically through either the left or right nostril activates different parts of the brain, and accesses different levels of consciousness. If this is true, it represents another opportunity for self-regulation. For the purpose of this exercise focus on the tip of your nose, and become aware of the temperature of the incoming and outgoing air. (pause one minute)

Imagine yourself as a small particle of air about to take an inward journey. You enter through the nose, are warmed by the moist and well-vasculated nasal tissues, and join the flow of air shaped by the sides of the inner nose, the nasal turbinates. The mucus of the nose touches and briefly sticks to you as it gently removes any undesirable contaminants. (pause two minutes)

You move through the upper nose and back down the throat for a sharp vertical drop through the throat, larynx, and trachea. Looking around, you can see the outside world through the opened mouth, the cartilage rings of the trachea, the thyroid gland pushing down upon the trachea, the fine little hairs, cilia, beating in rhythm and reminding you of the gentle and synchronous movements of a wheat field on a windy day. (pause two minutes)

When you reach the first branch of the trachea, you must make a decision to go right or left into either of the two main bronchi. You can feel the suction pulling you past the glistening moist lining of the breathing tree into smaller and smaller branches. (pause one minute) With each branching, the pull becomes stronger. Finally, you are released into the balloon-like opening of the alveoli. You have a few moments to look around, (pause one minute), and then you must offer your oxygen to the red blood cells that are awaiting you, ready to offer you the carbon dioxide that is needed by the plants. This transfer of nutrients connects inner and outer worlds. Feel this union, and the sharing of the food of life. (pause two minutes)

Soon it is time to leave, and you feel the pressure pushing you back up the canals of the trachea. With increasing force, you begin your journey up the trachea, and through the vibrating muscles of the larynx, which, if not for you, could not make their sounds. (pause one minute) One final look through the open mouth from the back of the throat, up through the nose, warmed by the membranes, through the tip of the nose and into the outer world. (pause one minute) Here you meet and mix with your fellow particles of air and continue your task as carrier of the world's energy. For a few moments, experience the sacredness of the act of breathing. (pause two minutes)

Return your focus to your mind. Is it still? What is the quality of your breathing? Is it soft, rhythmic, and gentle? Observe your breathing. (pause two minutes) Are you breathing from your chest muscles or diaphragm? If your mind is quiet, your breathing and body must also be quiet. Remain quiet and relaxed for several minutes. (pause five minutes)

It is now time to slowly open your eyes and reorient yourself to the time and space of the room.

Fortunately, breathing is predominantly an automatic process requiring minimal conscious attention. Increasing your awareness of breathing will, however, provide you with the 1) ability, however limited it may seem, to regulate the quality of the air you breathe, 2) capacity to use your breathing as a guide to your moment-to-moment levels of tension/relaxation, and 3) potential for using your breathing cycle to quiet your mind and rebalance your physiology. As you become increasingly attentive to your breathing by practicing the breathing exercises (see following exercise and breathing exercise in chapter 5), and checking on it during the day, you will discover an extraordinary built-in mechanism for self-regulating your mind and body. Awareness and control of your breathing can provide you with an essential ally in your quest for health.

EXERCISE 10:

CONTROLLED BREATHING (2)

Exercise 6 in chapter 5 introduced controlled breathing. These exercises emphasize self-regulation of breathing through the 1) conscious use of all the breathing muscles, 2) timing of inhalation and exhalation, and 3) controlling the internal and external space of breathing. The following exercise teaches another breathing technique, alternate nostril breathing. This technique is based on the yogic belief that at different times of the day we breathe predominantly through one or the other nostril, and that each nostril preferentially aerates a different part of the brain thereby activating a physiologic response characteristic of the specific nostril.

When practicing this exercise 1) continue your awareness of the breathing process, 2) observe whether you can identify a difference between right and left nostril breathing, and 3) again notice how working with your breath assists in shifting your mind to mindfulness. Begin this exercise by sitting in a chair in a manner described in Exercise 6. Allow thirty minutes. I would suggest first learning and practicing this technique from the text. If it is useful, you may then record it on an audiotape.

Sitting quietly with your eyes closed, take ten complete breaths, and then continue with diaphragmatic breathing. Curling the index and middle finger of the right hand, allow the thumb to rest on the right nostril and the index finger on the left. Your fingers will be used to close first one and then the other nostril.

Take a breath in through your left nostril while simultaneously occluding your right nostril with your right thumb. When the inhalation is complete switch nostrils by releasing the pressure and exhaling on the right while occluding the left nostril with your index finger. Let the air out through your right nostril and when complete take it back in through your right nostril and again switch sides for the next exhalation and inhalation.

Practice this sequence. (practice for five minutes) Next count from one to four during the inhalation and from one to eight for the exhalation, taking twice the time for exhalation as inhalation. (practice for ten minutes)

Next, focus on slowing the cycles. Maintain the same ratio of two to one between exhalation and inhalation, but slow the pace of the breathing and counting. Feel the body slow down with the breath. (practice for five minutes) Then, following inhalation, hold the breath for a count of four. The sequence will then be exhalation, inhalation, hold, exhalation, inhalation, hold—count eight, four, four, eight, four, four. (practice for five minutes)

Continue this for ten additional cycles. Become aware of the sensation of breathing through alternate nostrils. Notice the feeling in the body and the quieting that is possible through self-regulation of the breath.

Several times each day, stop for a moment, take several complete breaths, and then continue with diaphragmatic breathing. With practice, breathing techniques will rapidly reestablish balance in your respiratory system, which will, in turn, balance your mind-body.

When complete, open your eyes, survey your mind and body, and note any changes. Return to your routine daily activities.

The preceding exercise is a compliment to the breathing exercise in chapter 5. Each of these exercises should enhance awareness of your breathing cycle and its interrelationship with the mind and body. Choose the one that is most effective for you and return to it whenever possible. It can serve as a quick and effective way to quiet your mind and body, and assist you in gathering yourself back together when you feel scattered and distracted.

The following are additional practices that can assist you in regulating your respiratory system on a daily basis.

- Dairy products increase mucus production. By controlling dietary intake of dairy you can regulate mucus production.
- Proper humidification counteracts the harmful effects of dry air on the lining of the respiratory tract.
- Aerobic conditioning enables the body to maximize the use of oxygen from inhaled air while minimizing the energy involved in transferring the oxygen from the air to the blood system. It is important to understand how to properly condition your body and to be sure there are no reasons you should not perform such exercises (check with your physician).

- Diaphragmatic breathing will decrease the energy expenditure required for breathing.
- Minimizing your exposure to air pollutants will decrease mucus production and avoid damage to respiratory tissues.

THE CIRCULATORY SYSTEM

The circulatory system is the body's pickup and delivery system. Consisting of the heart, arteries, and veins, this system connects organ to organ, limb to limb, and brain to body. It delivers oxygen from the lungs and nutrients from the stomach and small intestine to the remainder of the body. Simultaneously, it retrieves the unneeded end products of metabolism and delivers them to the lungs, skin, and kidneys for excretion. The system moves hormones and other neuropeptides from their source in the glands and brain to appropriate sites in the body and transports the components of the immune system, which at all times are ready to go to where they are needed to defend against abnormal cells or bacterial and viral invaders.

The heart, which serves as the central pump, receives on its right side deoxygenated blood from the veins, which it sends directly to the lungs. Oxygenated blood returning from the lungs enters the left side of the heart, where it is forcefully pumped into the great blood vessels. The heart, an extraordinary muscle, pumps continuously at a baseline rate of eighty beats per minute. It is able to readjust to the changing needs of the body by slowing or accelerating its pace and diminishing or intensifying its contractual power. These readjustments are controlled by the autonomic nervous system and the stress-related hormone, adrenaline.

Upon leaving the heart, blood enters the arteries. The arteries are a series of branching tubes, whose central opening is surrounded by a lining called the mucosa, and several layers of muscle that contract in a synchronous serpentine manner, assisting the heart in moving blood through the system. Beginning with the largest artery, the aorta, the tubes slowly decrease their diameter as they move further from the heart until they reach the microscopic diameter of capillaries, where the actual exchange of nutrients between the circulatory system and the cells of the body takes place.

In a normal and healthy state, the mucosal lining of the arteries is smooth and compliant, and the muscles surrounding the mucosa are in a relaxed state, contracting only when necessary to move the blood. When the blood reaches the final small branches of the arterial system, the capillaries, it is ready for its return to the heart. It empties into the veins, which return blood from the body to the heart. Veins, although tubular like the arteries, are more like expandable sacs. Unlike the arteries, they are not muscular, and must rely on gravity, the contraction of adjacent muscles, and the critical placement of internal valves that prevent backsliding of the blood. After slowly taking the blood through the body, the veins release it to the right side of the heart. Left to its natural homeostatic balance, this marvelous circulatory system can last many decades.

THE BROKEN HEART

The two major diseases of the heart are hypertension and atherosclerosis. Hypertension, elevated pressure within the arteries, is the result of an excessive push of a stressed heart and/or the inelasticity of damaged arterial mucosa or overtense muscular arteries. It can lead to hemorrhage in the brain, commonly called a stroke, and direct damage to a variety of organs including the heart. Atherosclerosis, a destructive narrowing of the central passageway of the blood vessels, is caused by abnormal deposits of calcium and cholesterol-containing plaques. Atherosclerosis can diminish the blood supply to organs and result in tissue destruction. When this happens in the heart it is called a heart attack. Each of these conditions, hypertension and atherosclerosis, and their complications, can be prevented in part, or sometimes totally, through mindfulness and self-regulation.

Fewer than five percent of the cases of high blood pressure are caused by surgically correctable mechanical problems. All the other cases, termed "essential hypertension," result from the increased pumping action of the heart and excessive tone of the muscular arteries. The increased action is brought on when the autonomic nervous system and the hormones that control the muscular activity of the heart and arteries are activated by stress. The autonomic nervous system consists of two opposing sets of nerves, the sympathetic and parasympathetic. The former activates the heart, increasing its rate and intensity. The latter slows the circulation, decreasing the work of the heart. The sympathetic nervous system is activated by stress, the parasympathetic by relaxation.

Although there is a component of hypertension that is passed on genetically and is not under our direct control, the extent and degree to which this natural *tendency*, and its secondary complications of heart disease and stroke, becomes *reality* is under our control. It is well known that individuals with a tendency toward high blood pressure often elevate their blood pressure to abnormal ranges when visiting a physician. This has been called "white coat hypertension." It is also apparent that the stressful response to daily life events results in an activated mind, body, and blood pressure. As previously mentioned, Dr. Peter L. Schnall at the Cardiovascular and Hypertension Center, New York Hospital—Cornell Medical College has clearly demonstrated the relationship between job strain, high job demands with little control, on the development of acute and chronic high blood pressure. For these and other individuals the constantly activated mind and body is a way of life. Mindfulness and self-regulation can deal with hypertension at the source: unhealthy mind-styles and life-styles.

To sit such an individual in a chair, expand his or her awareness of the circulatory system through mindfulness practice, teach a relaxation technique, or train him or her with biofeedback, is to witness the capacity of individuals to become mindful of the state of the body and, with precision, self-regulate the circulatory system. There is now no doubt that if an individual wants to work hard enough and long enough, it is possible to maintain a normal blood pressure without medications. For those for whom the latter is not possible, they can at least significantly reduce the need for medications.

In atherosclerosis, beginning early in life, thick plaques containing calcium and cholesterol are deposited on the walls of the arteries, slowly occluding them and obstructing the flow of blood. When this occurs in the arteries feeding the heart, the result is destruction of the affected heart tissue. This is what we call a "heart attack," a curious term suggesting that our circulatory system is attacked from outside rather than by acknowledging the truth, that personal decisions or actions such as diet, smoking, or stressful situations directly affect the development of this disorder.

The three major risk factors for atherosclerotic heart disease are smoking, high blood pressure, and elevated levels of cholesterol. Highly publicized hypertension, cholesterol, and smoking programs have, in part, been responsible for the decreasing incidence of these diseases over the past twenty-five years, but these programs, however, are not enough. Many individuals continue to suffer atherosclerosis and hypertension requiring doctors and drugs to treat the end stages of these diseases. Yet these disorders are preventable through mindfulness and self-regulation: smoking can be stopped through personal choice, hypertension can be controlled through self-regulation and medication, and elevated cholesterol, except in cases of severe genetic disorders, can be controlled through diet. Although these simple self-regulatory practices are well known to us, many people do not practice them.

In addition to the regulation of blood pressure and the maintenance of a healthy heart and blood vessels, we can further self-regulate and optimize the efficiency of the cardiovascular system through conditioning of the heart. Like any other muscle, the heart can be strengthened with a structured program of aerobic conditioning. Sustained exertion that elevates the pulse to a specified percentage of its maximum rate for thirty minutes, three times each week will result in a conditioned heart. The conditioned heart is more efficient and requires less energy and work to provide the same amount of oxygen to the body. The baseline pulse is reduced, a set amount of work requires less activation of the heart, and the heart itself requires less blood.

Gerald T. O'Connor and his associates at the Brigham and Woman's Hospital reviewed the medical literature to evaluate the effects of rehabilitation exercise in individuals recovering from coronary heart disease. The research suggests that, even in a group of individuals suffering the end stages of this disease, exercise was able to reduce future mortality, as measured in the three years of this study, by up to twenty percent.

Cardiovascular conditioning is an excellent example of our capacity to self-regulate the body and define through our choices and actions the state of our body physiology. It is remarkable that the cardiovascular system, which is so easy to self-regulate, is the source of the highest rate of disability and premature death in our society. What is true for our society is not true for other societies whose diets are healthier and whose natural life-styles require strenuous physical activity.

The following exercise will assist you in becoming mindful of the circulatory system. Repeat it as many times as needed to develop a more precise mindfulness of the circulatory system. Extend this to your daily life noting when the heart is racing or pounding, and when your body feels "turned up." The more finely tuned your mindfulness, the more effectively you can self-regulate this system. Allow thirty minutes for this exercise, with frequent one minute pauses every few sentences.

EXERCISE 11:

THE CARDIOVASCULAR SYSTEM

Find a quiet spot, sit comfortably, and close your eyes. Begin with ten complete breaths. Now create an image of yourself as a red blood cell—small, round, red, and pliable. You are capable of molding your shape to the inner channel of the blood vessels and are durable enough to withstand the regular push of the heart. As a red blood cell, consider yourself gifted with the capacity for "heartfulness," your task in life is to serve your community by delivering nourishment to all the cells of the body and removing the leftovers of metabolism.

You are born in the bone marrow. This cavern of darkness is situated in the central core of the long bones of the body, which protect your infancy with their strength. This is also the birthplace of the platelets and white blood cells. When you have reached maturity, and only then, you are released into the blood circulation. Suddenly, for the first time, you are swept up in the movement of the fluid blood, and soon find yourself in the large right chamber of the heart. You stop for a moment to look around at the first sac you enter—the right atrium. The surface is smooth and glistening. It is a place of rest.

Much to your surprise, suddenly, you fall through a narrow opening, the valve that separates the right atrial sac from the more powerful right ventricle. The ventricle is larger, and forcefully contracts and expands every few seconds. At times it beats faster and at times slower. With one of these beats you are propelled into the large pulmonary arteries, and discover yourself in an increasingly narrower tube, until you enter the small cramped capillaries of the alveoli, the air-containing sacs

of the lungs. To move through these capillaries you must bend
and mold yourself to their shape. Only a thin layer separates you
from the outer world, which reaches you through the inhaled air
of the lungs, but you remain at your task, serving the inner
world of the body.

While in the alveoli, you notice some chemical reactions
taking place in your body. A substance of yours called
hemoglobin is accepting oxygen from the inhaled air and giving
back any carbon dioxide you picked up in your first run through
the body. You fall back into the left atrial sac of the heart and
drop through the valve that separates this chamber from the
powerful left ventricle, which, with the next contraction,
strongly propels you into the largest artery of the body, the
aorta.

As you enter the aorta, you immediately see on your left and
right the small openings to the coronary blood vessels, the
arteries that nourish the heart. You and your fellow cells know
that without a healthy heart, without caring for the source of
your strength, your task will never be accomplished. Some of
your fellow travelers are honored to feed the heart by passing
into the coronary arteries. The remainder continue their journey
through the circulatory system.

There are many stop off points and reroutings possible on
your journey through the arteries and veins. As you move along
you can see the entrances to the arteries that serve the skin,
nerves, kidneys, liver, intestines, and all the other organs and
tissues of the body. A red blood cell has to be flexible and learn
many chores. You pick up nutrients from the small intestine,
drop off unnecessary waste products at the kidneys, pick up
hormones from the glands, distribute nutrients and hormones
throughout the body, and warm the skin. You can feel the
arteries contracting their muscles to provide an extra push as
you get farther and farther from the heart.

While traveling through the blood vessels, you may run into a
blockage, which stops your smooth flowing journey. The smooth
silky container of your life is disrupted by a rough section of
hard, jagged, and irregular cholesterol deposits that scratch your
skin, bump you around, and, at times, force you to squeeze

yourself as small as possible to get by. It may be necessary for you to forego your rounds, taking a detour around the occluded and destroyed blood vessels. The tissues that you cannot nourish will grow unhealthy and deteriorate.

Soon you enter the saclike veins. This is a time for rest before your next trip through the arteries. Slowly, you make your way back to the right side of the heart, joined by the many other cells, who have taken a different route. Lacking oxygen and filled with carbon dioxide, your color is a bit more blue than red. Back you fall into the heart, ready to return to service for another trip through the body—a life of travel that will continue for 120 days of a human life, the lifespan of a red blood cell.

When finished, slowly open your eyes and return to the time and space of the room.

Atheroslcerotic plaques are present on the blood vessels walls of many young adults, as was observed in autopsies of young soldiers who died in the Korean war. There is increasing evidence that in our culture these plaques begin to develop at a very young age. Because this deterioration of the normal integrity and patency of our blood vessels is unfortunately almost "normal" among westerners, I have included these changes in the imagery exercise to sensitize each of us to their presence. As previously discussed in this chapter, these changes are not normal and they are reversible through self-regulation.

The following list summarizes practices that can assist in self-regulating the circulatory system.

- Reduce the intake of salt
- Reduce the intake of animal products (meat, dairy, and eggs), which provide cholesterol and saturated fats
- Regularly engage in aerobic cardiovascular conditioning
- Do not smoke
- Practice the daily mindfulness training exercise as a way of regulating a hyperactive and "agitated" circulation.
- Consider biofeedback training to self-regulate elevated blood pressure
- Cultivate a life of contentment

Mindfulness, accompanied by the regular use of self-regulatory techniques, can provide you with an extraordinary capacity to control and favorably influence many aspects of the circulatory system previously thought to be uncontrollable through conscious decisions and actions. The great epidemic of heart disease is largely preventable through these simple techniques. If there is any remaining doubt about our capacity to self-regulate atherosclerotic heart disease, it can be quickly eliminated by a look at the statistics. From the 1960s to the present date we have seen a remarkable decline in deaths from heart disease. This decline exceeds fifty percent in younger age groups and approaches that figure in older age groups. The reasons: regulation of blood pressure, decreases in smoking, diminished intake of fats, more exercise, and improved treatment techniques.

THE GASTROINTESTINAL SYSTEM

The gastrointestinal (GI) system, like the respiratory system, is a direct connection with the outside world. From the opening of the mouth, through the esophagus, stomach, and small and large intestines, the outer world flows through the center of our body. The interface between ourselves and the external environment is a thin layer of sensitive tissue, the mucosa, that lines our GI system.

Transforming food from the outer world into the energy and material of the body begins with the specific food we consciously choose from the many possible sources of food. When we eat, digestive juices are released in the mouth, and, by the chopping action of our teeth, food is partially digested and prepared for further chemical breakdown in the stomach. Propelled by the musculature of the mouth, and assisted by the synchronous and rhythmic contractions of the esophageal muscles, partially digested food flows down the esophagus and through a door, the esophageal sphincter, that opens into the stomach.

The lining of the stomach contains specialized cells that excrete additional digestive chemicals. Slowly, in this mixture of enzymes, acid, and food, our GI system extracts the body's nourishment. The chemical constituents of ingested food, the microchemical constituents of life, are soon ready for absorption into the small capillaries underneath the mucosal lining of the stomach. The mucosa carefully chooses what it will take from the outside world and sends the remaining undigested food to the small intestine, through the next door, the pyloric sphincter.

The small intestine has three sections, the duodenum, jejunum, and ileum. These receive digestive juices from the pancreas and continue the process of digestion and absorption, passing appropriate micronutrients into the waiting blood stream and routing the remainder to the large intestine through the propelling force of its muscular contractions. The process of digestion is completed in the small intestine.

Any remaining unabsorbable food is joined in the large intestine by the unneeded end products of metabolism and is ultimately excreted through the anus. The large intestine, encircled by muscle, contracts in a coordinated serpentine manner to move the excrement out of the body in an orderly and timely fashion. This completes one cycle of a continuous process of digestion. In the normal functioning of this system, we are able to take in what we need and let go of what is unusable. When the GI system is cared for, its natural process of homeostasis maintains a healthy and balanced digestive process. Too often this is not the case.

THE UPSET STOMACH

The mucosal lining of the GI system is exceedingly sensitive to both the content of ingested food and shifts in our emotions. It is tolerant, but its tolerance, which is severely tested in our culture, is not without limits. The major disorders of this system, gastritis, duodenal ulcer disease, Crohn's disease, ulcerative colitis, diverticulosis, and colon cancer are related to the content of our food and the stress in our lives.

Our GI system, which was once limited to the day's capture and harvest and accustomed to natural and untainted foods, must now be on the defensive. Rather than joyfully greeting the outer world, it must cope with unhealthy chemicals, food that comes from factories rather than fields, inadequate amounts of clean water, and internal disorder caused by the chemicals and hormones that are released within the body at times of stress. Homeostasis is difficult to achieve under these circumstances.

The expressions "butterfly in my stomach," "nervous stomach," and "gut feeling" reflect the well known reactivity of the stomach to stress and distress. The lining of the bowel, the mucosa, is rich in neuropeptide receptors. The bridge between the receptors and the emotional centers of the brain is the flow of neuropeptides, the brain chemicals that act as messengers transforming any mental distress into a distressed GI system. Stress and intense emotions release these chemicals that disrupt the normal integrity of the stomach surface, creating an increased susceptibility to the erosive actions of the gastric digestive juices, which begin to "digest" the stomach instead of food. The symptoms of disordered gastric digestion, ranging from brief periods of nausea, bloating, gaseousness, and stomach distress, to the full scale emergency of a bleeding ulcer, result from the unchecked corrosive action of these internal chemicals often assisted by alcohol, aspirin, and a variety of other natural and man-made chemicals that further disorder stomach digestion.

As we move down the GI system, the effects of stress and the sensitivity of this system to emotional distress become even more apparent. Crohn's disease and ulcerative colitis, two examples of the intimate connection between the bowel and stress, are disorders caused by both genetic and personal factors. Although the genetic factors are not under our control, the degree to which the genetic tendency becomes manifest as actual disease can be significantly affected by mind-style and life-style. Individuals suffering from these disorders can frequently associate exacerbations and remissions of disease with the emergence and disappearance of stress.

Colon cancer, a common form of cancer in both men and women, has an increased incidence in members of the same family. This disease is ten times more prevalent in Western countries than in Far Eastern and developing countries. It has been suggested by researchers that up to ninty percent of the variation between countries is related to the differences in consumption of animal fats. Observing two simple dietary rules, 1) eating moderate amounts of fiber and 2) reducing the intake of fats, may markedly reduce the risk of colon cancer. Using only natural and whole foods can also reduce any further unknown influences from chemical toxins, insecticides, additives, and preservatives.

Two less serious but disturbing disorders of the large intestine are irritable bowel syndrome, also called spastic colitis, and diverticulosis. Irritable bowel syndrome is a disorder of the muscular contractions of the large bowel causing abdominal pain, accompanied by alternating diarrhea and constipation. This disorder is significantly associated with stress, and, for the individual willing to make substantive life changes, it can be quite responsive to self-regulation.

Diverticulosis, small outpocketings of the walls of the lower intestine, is thought to be similarly caused by disordered muscular contractions, which is, in part, related to the amount of fiber that is ingested in our diet. This disorder takes many years to develop, often manifesting in later life with a painful and distressing infection called diverticulitis.

Working with individuals with these disorders, I always emphasize continuing the important, and frequently helpful, medical treatments, and the necessity of making significant and long-term life changes. The latter is the only possible permanent solution to these chronic disorders. Often the question that must be answered is, "Do I prefer the disease, or do I prefer making difficult and substantial changes in my life?" It is rarely possible to continue the same life-style, and at the same time minimize or heal these diseases. Although many of these disorders are responsive to self-regulation, healing is not instantaneous. Just as there is a lag period between the onset of stress and the development of overt illness, there is also a lag between life-style changes, and the healing of a disorder.

These disorders, and the drugs used to relieve them, are responsible for a large percentage of physician office visits and prescriptions, respectively. Although treatments for these disorders, which temporarily relieve symptoms, are abundant, the potential for permanent healing through the use of mindfulness and self-regulatory techniques is only rarely considered (Refer back to "John's story" in chapter 1 and 2. His healing is one of many I have seen in individuals who are willing to commit themselves to nonpharmacologic approaches to stress-related disorders of the GI system.). Because these disorders are not so "glamorous" or fatal as coronary heart disease, there has yet to be significant scientific research documenting the capacity to self-regulate and heal these disorders. Yet the role of the mind in the development, activation, and progression of these disorders is apparent to both those who suffer from these disorders and those who care for them. Failure to recognize this fact and resolve the underlying causes of GI disorders results in continued physiologic imbalance and contributes to the perpetuation of these diseases.

The GI system is a wonderful source of life. Too often it is a source of

distress. Through mindfulness and self-regulatory practices we can discover the unhealthy inner attitudes that too frequently express
themselves through this system and the self-healing attitudes and actions that result in a healthy mind and body. We no longer have the
false luxury of exclusively looking outside of ourselves for explanations
and treatments to these disorders. We are each capable of maintaining
the balance of this interface between outer and inner world, mind and
body, thus promoting health, and avoiding unnecessary disease.

For the following exercise refer to the instructions for Exercise 9.
Allow thirty minutes for this exercise with one minute pauses every few
sentences.

EXERCISE 12:
_____

THE GASTROINTESTINAL SYSTEM

Sit comfortably in a chair, close your eyes, take five complete
breaths, and begin this exercise. Imagine a piece of food, your
favorite vegetable, placed in front of you. As a vegetable, it is
grown from the soil, matured by the sun, and picked as an
offering to the human life cycle. It is life giving to life. If you
are lucky, its birth and growth have been natural. It has been
untainted by chemicals and picked at the moment of its
sweetness.

Its mission is to nourish others, as the soil, sun, and rain have
nourished it. It has been washed, sliced into digestible
segments, and finally honored for the life it conveys. Its first
contact with the human body is the mouth. In this warm
container, it is slowly prepared for further digestion through the
chewing actions of the teeth and digestive juices of the mouth.
For the next two minutes that it remains in the mouth,
experience its warmth and its slow return to its basic chemical
parts.

When it is well prepared, and only then, the food is
swallowed for a ride down the esophagus, which, with its
rhythmic contractions, gently pushes the food into the waiting
stomach. Now it is more of a paste. As it is further broken into

its chemical constituents, it is absorbed into the blood for distribution to the body, and other parts are shunted to the small intestine for further digestion. At all times, there is movement and activity around it. What remains of it reaches the large intestine. The movement is slower as its undigestible parts are compacted, given back to the earth.

It becomes incorporated into the tissues and cells of the body and serves many purposes: It provides protein for the building blocks of cells, sugar as a source of energy, fat as a source of stored energy, and is used as a building block for important body chemicals. Inevitably it, as all else, will be returned to the earth. As it has been transformed from seed to plant to human, so also in the form of a human will it return to soil, plant, and seed. It, like the air, is another movement of the earth and universe through our body.

Remain for several minutes in quiet reverence of this continuously transforming universe and the magnificent role of the GI system in providing for your sustenance.

When finished, slowly return your awareness to the room.

It is important to expand your awareness of this system through your daily life experiences. Become increasingly observant of your food choices, eating patterns, and any related discomfort in your stomach or bowels. Observe how this system is influenced by your moods, size of your meal, pace of your meal, the setting in which you eat, the people you eat with, the manner in which your food is prepared, the distribution of proteins, carbohydrates, and fats in your food, and the presence of additives and other chemicals. It is important to inquire even further and more precisely determine the relationship of your life to the operation of your GI system. There is no reason why your body, particularly this system, should be a stranger to you. The more you know, the more and better choices you can make.

The following list summarizes practices that may assist you in regulating your bowels.

- Emphasize carbohydrates, fiber, and unprocessed foods, which are foods that have taken a minimal detour from the farm to your grocery store

- Minimize animal fats
- Drink lots of water
- Have modest-sized meals that you chew and eat slowly with mind-fulness
- Practice the daily mindfulness training exercise
- If appropriate, consider biofeedback training to assist with relaxation

THE IMMUNE SYSTEM

The immune system is our natural defense against bacteria, viruses, and the proliferation of abnormal cancerous cells. It is a constantly moving system. Unlike previous systems we have discussed, this system is mobile and circulates throughout the body via the arteries and veins. It is composed of many different specialized cells that interact in ways that we are only beginning to understand. The available information on this system is quickly accumulating in response to rapidly advancing research on cancer and Acquired Immunodeficiency Syndrome (AIDS).

The operating immune system is a marvel. It is able to tell the difference between cells and chemicals belonging to the body and those that are foreign to it. In addition to this sensitivity and specificity, the system's built-in memory can recall after an initial contact with a foreign invader the chemical label of the specific foreign substance. This recall is the basis of immunity and immunization.

The system operates in three fundamental ways (see Figure 6.1). The first is called T cell mediated immunity. In this form of immunity a specific set of cells identify and directly lead an attack of cells on "invaders" and inform other active components of the immune system of the impending danger. The second strategy relies on cells called B cells. This approach, also called humoral antibody immunity, uses chemicals called antibodies that circulate in the blood and quickly attack invading bacteria or viruses. The third strategy relies on a group of cells called natural killer cells, which do not require presensitization or previous contact with a foreign invader to attack and immobilize it.

T cell immunity	There are two subsets of T cells: helper and suppressor. The helper cells directly attack the invaders and stimulate the B cells to produce antibodies. The suppressor cells suppress the immune response.
B cell immunity	The B cells produce specific antibodies that destroy foreign invaders. These cells have a memory, which allows them to respond immediately to and recognize the foreign invader if it reappears in the future.
Natural killer cells	This group of large cells can attack and destroy a variety of bacteria, viruses, and abnormal cells without prior sensitization.

Figure 6.1. The immune system.

Cell mediated immunity relies on a type of white blood cell called the T cell. The T cells migrate from the bone marrow to the thymus gland, a small gland situated under the breast bone, where they mature to adult, fully functional T cells. There are several different types of T cells: Helper T cells facilitate the defensive action of other immune cells, suppressor T cells dampen the action of the immune system, and killer T cells, which, when previously exposed to an abnormal virus or cancerous cell, destroy the invader on recontact. Helper and suppressor T cells function by releasing chemical messengers called lymphokines, which "talk" to the other parts of the immune system.

Antibody mediated immunity relies on another type of white blood cell called the B cell. The B cells do not directly attack an invader. When they become aware of one, they multiply and produce chemicals called antibodies, which differ according to the specific type of invader. An antibody attaches to and destroys the invader. This rapidly acting system is a complement to the slower acting cell mediated immunity.

The third approach relies on a type of cell called the natural killer cell. This cell, which is actually a subtype of T cell, is viewed as a separate system because it does not require initial contact with the foreign invader to "gear it up" for attack. The natural killer cells, the third system, support cell mediated and immune mediated immunity and, through their capacity to respond directly and immediately to abnormal cells and destroy them may be central to the prevention of cancer. The entire immune system, containing these three subsystems, is at all times circulating in our blood vessels, protecting and defending the integrity of our mind and body.

When less was known about this system, it was thought to be preprogrammed, acting autonomously, independent of other organ systems, and not subject to voluntary control or self-regulation. As we learn more about this extraordinary invention of nature, we increasingly recognize its capacity to interact with all aspects of the mind and body and its susceptibility to self-regulation. When the system is healthy and in homeostatic balance, it protects us against an array of bacteria, viruses, and the continuous low-level emergence of abnormal and cancerous cells. When the system is in disorder, the results are catastrophic.

DISORDERED IMMUNITY

In 1981, an unusual disease appeared in a young man. This disease, Kaposi's sarcoma, is rare and infrequently affects young men. Less than a decade later, with thousands afflicted and dying, we have come to know this disease of disordered immunity as AIDS. This disease results from the destructive effect of a certain virus (HTLV-3) on helper T cells. The immune system, without this major component, is incapable of defending itself against foreign invaders and abnormal cell growth. This impairment of the immune system leaves the body undefended.

A second major disorder of the immune system is its loss of sensitivity to the difference between cells that are normal to the body, and cells that are abnormal. Our body, as a part of its normal breakdown of aging cells and regeneration of new cells, routinely produces abnormal cancerous cells. The immune system quickly destroys these cells and removes them from circulation. In certain instances, for reasons still poorly understood, the immune system loses its capacity to identify these abnormal cells, allowing them to grow uncontrollably into cancer.

A major direction in cancer research and therapy has been the development of increasingly sophisticated techniques to destroy abnormal cells through the use of toxic pharmaceuticals or radiation treatments. This effort is now being expanded to include the use of mind-body self-regulating techniques, including meditation, guided imagery, biofeedback, and attitudinal healing. These techniques, directed toward strengthening the immune system, offer the enormous potential of using the relatively untapped natural healing capacities of the mind-body. Although, as of this date, they lack full scientific validation, it is expected that the rapidly expanding research in PNI will document and define the pathways through which these techniques assist in enhancing the efficacy of the immune system.

A third disorder of the immune system occurs when the body fails to recognize its own cells and begins to attack itself, destroying its own tissues. These disorders, called autoimmune diseases, include arthritis, systemic lupus, Hashimoto's thyroid disease, and vasculitis, among numerous other such disorders. In these disturbances, the aim of medical therapy is to reduce the potency of the immune system. Unfortunately, this cannot be done specifically for the tissues at risk. Therefore, the treatment itself frequently places the individual at risk for other invaders.

We know that homeostasis is essential for the healthy functioning of the immune system. We are beginning to understand, learn, and practice techniques that will expand our capacity to self-regulate what we previously believed to be a fully automatic system not amenable to conscious regulation. Like the other body systems, immune system disorders are often the result of predisposing factors. As an example, our genetic inheritance predisposes some of us to develop certain diseases and forms of cancer. The genetic predisposition may, however, be insufficient to cause actual disease. As is true of the other systems, the pivotal factors in determining whether these tendencies become actual disease are our mind-style and life-style.

The foods we eat, the thoughts we hold, the images we see, and our stress levels are directly related to the functioning of our immune system. This is the most exciting part of the story. For example, health care providers who visit their patients regularly know that a winter virus that moves through the community does not affect all individuals equally. Those who are most stressed and fatigued succumb first and take the longest to recover. As physicians, we are also aware of the strong, although as yet unproven, impression that cancer develops in individuals who live through persistent periods of depression and that individuals who lose a spouse have a considerably higher rate of illness and death in the year following the death. These and other observations lead us to new and innovative approaches to healing and rebalancing the disordered immune system through mindfulness and self-regulation.

Research has focused on the impact of certain attitudes and life perspectives on the immune system. Stress, discussed in chapter 6, and the mental attitudes of powerlessness, loneliness, and deprivation, discussed in chapter 7, are examples of how life-style and mind-style can suppress the immune system and diminish its capacity as a natural defense system. Growing out of this research are early efforts to intervene and self-regulate the immune system, among them relaxation techniques, particularly mindfulness training, mental imagery, various forms of psychotherapy, physical conditioning, and nutrition.

The following exercise will assist you in enhancing your understanding and awareness of the immune system. Because we cannot see, touch, or feel it as it works within our body, it is difficult to develop a direct mindfulness of this system. We can however become indirectly mindful of it by watching its results in our daily life, our susceptibility to infections, and by becoming mindful of the conditions, as an example stress, that suppress the system. Allow thirty minutes for this exercise with one minute pauses every few sentences.

EXERCISE 13:

THE IMMUNE SYSTEM

Sit comfortably in a chair, close your eyes, and begin this exercise. Imagine yourself to be a white cell. For this exercise, become a helper T cell, the white blood cell that matures in the thymus gland and is the main source of cell mediated immunity. You are circulating within the bloodstream in the company of the red blood cells and the micronutrients absorbed from the gastrointestinal system.

Your job, unlike that of the B cell which tends to remain in the area of lymph nodes and lymphoid-like tissue, is to move throughout the body, seeking out and destroying abnormal cells, bacteria, or viruses, and informing the B cells of the presence of invaders. You may spend many hours with little to do except standing guard. Suddenly, a bacterial invader moves against your surface, or you are warned of the presence of invaders by a special warning cell called a macrophage. You identify the invader by its specific chemical label and send out a chemical signal to the killer T cells, which then surround the bacteria and destroy it.

While you are busy with this, you also call on the B cells to produce antibodies, which also seek out the invaders and destroy them. Soon, the scavenger macrophages arrive on the scene and with the killer T cells, surround and do battle with the bacteria.

Assuming the immune system is healthy, you will win this battle. As a result, there will be a new set of T and B cells that now will remember the chemical label of this foreign invader and stand guard against its reappearance, ready to respond quickly.

The excitement over, you return again to your task of surveillance. For long periods of time this may seem unworthy of your attention, but you are aware that the continued health of the body depends on your presence. Perhaps you are surprised, given your importance, that from time to time, when the pressure of the blood increases, stress-related chemicals are released into the blood-stream. These diminish your power and preparedness and disorder your function. At other times, you notice that the body seems to be relaxed and in balance, which allows you to feel fully alive and capable of responding and reacting to any and all crises.

While you are circulating and standing guard, you may pass one of your cousins, a B cell, leisurely staying "home" in a lymph node or other lymphoid tissue such as the spleen. B cells screen the blood, moving through the lymph system for invaders, which, if found, are attacked and destroyed. During these battles the lymph node swells and becomes tender to external touch, giving us what we call "swollen glands."

As a cell in the immune system you are part of a two-way communication with the brain, using specific chemical messengers, called neuropeptides. Neuropeptides released by the immune cell reach the brain, warning it about the presence of foreign invaders. The brain mobilizes the other body systems to help defend the body's integrity by releasing its own neuropeptides. When they reach you, the helper T cell, they influence your health-sustaining actions. This two-way communication system allows you to respond to emotions arising in the brain through mental stress and allows the brain and emotions to respond to changes in the body's physiology as detected by you and other members of your immune system. In this manner, the immune system stays in constant contact with the mind and body.

It is now time to leave this system. Slowly open your eyes and return your awareness to the immediate surroundings of the room.

We can directly observe our breathing, study our GI system in action, and measure our pulse and blood pressure. The immune system is, however, more hidden from our view, and we are, thereby, separated and "estranged" from this essential aspect of our being. The above exercise is designed to place you in greater contact with this system, and allow you to feel its vitality, its service to you, and its interconnectedness with every other aspect of the mind and body. The closer you are to it and the more you know about how it works, the more you can "own" and work with it.

SELF-REGULATING THE IMMUNE SYSTEM

The capacity to self-regulate the immune system, the body's most important natural defense, is the power to prevent and heal disease. While PNI is slowly guiding us in the proper direction, innovative healing programs are already exploring the leading edges of self-regulatory healing. The following, some of which have been mentioned in previous chapters, are the technologies that have emerged from research in PNI and new medical approaches to strengthening the immune system:

Relaxation

Any healing program, particularly one that emphasizes self-regulation of the immune system, must include relaxation as its most important strategy. Mental and physiologic relaxation counteracts the suppression of the immune system caused by stress and the stress hormones: corticosteroids, epinephrine, and norepinephrine. When practiced on a regular basis, relaxation techniques reduce an individual's susceptibility to stress and, at the same time, minimize the effects of existing stress. The following approaches, all of which have been described in earlier chapters, can be used to self-regulate the immune system by inducing the relaxed state or assisting in eradicating the sources of stress: mindfulness training exercise, biofeedback, relaxation exercises, controlled breathing, guided imagery, and Hatha yoga.

Exercise

Exercise can regulate the immune system through its capacity to 1) reduce stress, 2) prevent or lessen depression, 3) stabilize a tendency for hyperactivation of the sympathetic nervous system (see chapter 2), and 4) activate brain centers that produce and release neuropeptides. Endorphins are the best known of these neuropeptides.

Some evidence also shows that an effect of heavy aerobic exercise may be the immediate and lingering activation of the immune system, which enhances its capacity for surveillance and the destruction of abnormal cells, bacteria, and viruses.

We have long known that exercise improves our general state of well being. What is new is the discovery of the pathways through which exercise enhances the hardiness of our immune system and the recognition that exercise, a chosen activity, can be used to self-regulate immunity.

Guided Imagery

Guided imagery has become a standard technique of innovative cancer treatment programs. Its goal is to enhance and maximize the immune system's response to cancerous cells. An individual with cancer enters a state of relaxation, then imagines, using mental imagery and other thoughts, the destruction of cancerous cells and the healing of the body.

Although there is insufficient scientific information to establish definitively the capacity of imagery to enhance the function of the immune system, there can be little doubt about the capacity of imagery to affect the physiology of the body. Imagine a wonderful French pastry or an erotic scene, for instance, and observe the effects these images have on your body. It is quite conceivable that we can use the power of imagery to self-regulate the immune system consciously.

The effect of imagery in inducing relaxation, deactivating the sympathetic nervous system, providing the individual with a renewed sense of control and power, and affecting the immune system, are the aspects of this technique that may assist in healing and prevention.

Attitudinal Healing

In chapter 7, we will review the effects of perceived powerlessness, loneliness, and deprivation on the body and specifically on the immune system. The research in PNI, although not definitive, suggests that shifts in these perspectives may enhance the function of the immune system through a reduction in stress and depression and potentially through directly enhancing the action of the immune system.

The many cognitive and experiential approaches to attitudinal healing include psychotherapy and assertiveness and communication training. In addition, this book describes and recommends the two-part approach of mindfulness and self-regulation as described in chapter 7.

Nutrition

Although there is much that should be said for the role of nutrition in regulating the immune system, because of the lack of research little can be said. We have discovered some chemicals, some natural and others synthesized, that affect the immune system. Many chemicals in our food may also have a natural capacity to inhibit or enhance the function of the immune system. It will require future research to provide us with an organized approach to self-regulation through our diet.

The small amount of available information suggests that elevated fats and obesity (or either condition separately) act to suppress the immune system, and yellow and orange vegetables serve to enhance the immune system. The former may, in part, explain the increased risk of cancer related to high intake of nutritional fats.

Sleep Deprivation and Social Support

We are likely to discover many other actions we can take to extend our capacity to self-regulate the immune system. For example, we now have evidence to suggest that among these, a good night's sleep and a healthy network of friends and loved ones can enhance the function of the immune system. Although the specific physiologic pathways are yet unclear, their effect on enhancing immune function is likely a result of an increased hardiness and resistance to stress and depression.

Conclusion

This chapter has reviewed the body's major organ systems in order to help you learn how mindfulness and self-regulation can be used to promote health and prevent illness. Setting aside the time necessary to work with the mindfulness exercises, and becoming mindful of the body as it functions on a day-to-day basis is the only way to fine tune your awareness and apply appropriate and timely self-regulation. The practices described in this chapter will assist you with this goal. It is important, however, to evaluate *your* body and its unique needs carefully. This can only be accomplished through a precise understanding of how your body works.

Chapter 7

REGULATING THE MIND

IN THE PRECEDING two chapters, we learned about the first two categories of self-regulation, general relaxation and regulating the body. In this chapter we will learn about regulating the mind. We will take a close look at three very common unhealthy and disease-inducing attitudes, powerlessness, loneliness, and deprivation, and examine how, using these as examples, the two components of self-regulation, conscious living and daily practices, can help us remember and re-experience the vitality, confidence, trust, and connectedness that each of us knew and lived before our minds were distorted and abused by the unhealthy attitudes and actions of immature adults.

The mind is an extraordinary, and, at times, it seems to be a somewhat strange creation. Left to itself it will recall and repeat what it has learned, however false and destructive this may be, rather than remember its natural and untainted gifts. With great courage and determination, it is possible to break through the barriers and boundaries imposed upon our lives by the biology of our brains and the ignorance of our early teachers. We can replace our misconceived perspectives with a knowledge that is authentic, personal, and enriching. We can use our mechanical, habit-forming minds to supplant unhealthy programs with healthy ones (we call this process conscious living) and use mindfulness to discover directly the truth of our lives. The truth invariably conveys with it a profound personal understanding that disempowers the misperceptions that force us to act in a manner inconsistent with our health. In this way we can reclaim from our parents, teachers, professionals, and society our responsibility and right to self-determine and self-direct the character and content of our mental life. Only then can we re-own and mature our birthright: the capacity for full health.

CONSCIOUS LIVING

Conscious living relies on and uses the built-in capacity of the mind to establish new habits when it is repetitively exposed to new behaviors. It allows us to reprogram our minds according to our view of life. Conscious living is an important first step toward regulating the mind and creating a healthy life. The incorporation into our daily lives of a basic set of important life-enhancing attitudes creates the context in which we can, with greater success and ease, regulate and change the more intractable and unhealthy aspects of our mind-talk. We can begin even if we are not quite there yet by acting as if we already had integrated these new attitudes. The following are examples of healthy conscious living:

BALANCE

Balance results from avoiding the extremes of behavior and maintaining a life-style that is harmonious and in synchrony with one's environment. It often requires self-restraint. Attention to the presence of mental and physical stress will enable the initiation of appropriate and timely actions that restore a feeling of balance. As an example, you may look at the proportion of time spent in outer activities to time spent in solitude. Is it appropriate for you? Does it help in maintaining a high level of well-being?

CONTENTMENT

Contentment results from a mental attitude that finds satisfaction in what is given in life. Contentment does not imply that we cease working for the visions and goals we choose for the future but that we are patient with our development, enjoy each day, and do not become absorbed in the moment-to-moment ups and downs of our efforts. The yogis state, ". . . happiness can be derived from contentment and not from thinking that I shall be happy when I get all I wish for."

SIMPLICITY

Simplicity is knowing the difference between what we want and what we need. Everything we possess, in a manner, possesses us. The yogis state it in this way, "There is trouble in acquiring objects which give us pleasure and enjoyment, trouble again in trying to preserve them and unhappiness when we lose them." The simpler we can make our lives, the less mental turmoil we will cause ourselves. We already have enough mind-talk—we do not need to add more.

HONESTY

Honesty is the cultivation of truth in our words. The yogis say it is "the correspondence of speech and mind to fact." They also suggest that, to cultivate truth, one should initially "speak as little as possible or observe silence." Honesty does not mean that everything must be said. It means that we must use discrimination when we put into words information that may cause harm rather than good.

HARMLESSNESS

It is important to abstain from actions and words that may be harmful to others. Harm can result not only from those things we do, but from necessary actions that we forego. Harmlessness also implies the cultivation of feelings of good will towards others and the relinquishing of harmful attitudes and behaviors such as greed, envy, and careless actions.

SOLITUDE

The importance of solitude has been discussed in chapter 3. It is essential to remember that solitude is not isolation or withdrawal. It is not avoidance or protection from the outer issues of life. Not unlike going to the beach for swimming, or to others for companionship and relationship, we must go in to ourselves to discover the truths of our life, heal our minds and bodies, "grow" our lives, and nurture and express our creativity.

This list is not meant to be complete. These attitudes and their related life-styles, along with others, result in a quieter mind, and a minimum of emotional and physical stress. Even when our minds have not yet developed to the point that these attitudes and practices are natural and spontaneous, we can use them as guidelines. They represent a conscious commitment to self-healing, helping to shape and regulate the development of a healthier mind. Do not attempt to incorporate them into your life all at once. Decide what is achievable and begin with small changes: perhaps attention to one change a month. Practice it daily, examine any resistance to it that may arise, observe any related changes that result from this new practice, and carefully cultivate its presence in your life.

MINDFULNESS AS SELF-REGULATION

The remainder of this chapter will examine three specific and common types of unhealthy mind talk: 1) powerlessness, which is experienced as helplessness and inadequacy, 2) loneliness, which is experienced as isolation, and 3) deprivation, which is experienced as continuously having unmet needs. In each of these situations, unhealthy psychologic mind-talk is exclusively responsible for emotional distress, fear, worry, and anxiety. However impossible it may seem to you (as we will discover, feeling "stuck" is a form of the attitude of powerlessness), you can move permanently beyond these attitudes to a sense of confidence and competence, connectedness and abundance. We cannot accomplish this through our intellect and analytic thinking. We must use a finely developed mindfulness.

In contrast to the intuitiveness of mindfulness, the analytic intellect gathers together many pieces of information and forms them into ideas and concepts. These ideas and concepts, stored in our memories and recollected as thoughts, serve as templates and guides that enable us to interpret and understand our experiences. Like the shadows of figures in Plato's "Allegory of the Cave" in *The Republic*, our ideas and concepts provide us with an indirect, superficial, and often inaccurate under-standing. This way of understanding, through our intellect and its thinking process, is often the source of our troubles and serves as a strong and almost impenetrable barrier to a more comprehensive, un-changing, and truthful understanding, which invariably releases us from the distress of misunderstandings and partial understandings.

The concentration of mindfulness provides us with another way of understanding. It allows us to break through the barriers of intellectual thinking and penetrate directly into our experiences in a way that provides us with an essential understanding that is often difficult to express in words. The intelligence of mindfulness is called creative intelligence. When we understand in this way we "know that we know" and have the feeling of the fit of a finely tailored garment. Such understanding is indivisible. It is fundamental and enduring; it has no shades or colors and does not lend itself to further analysis, judgment, or evaluation. It is what it is. It unbinds the anxious energy tied up with misperceptions and frees us to act.

To access this way of understanding, we must first move through the intellectual mind and become mindful. This is done by quieting mind-talk through attention. The quiet mind can then concentrate on an issue or problem it wishes to penetrate through in order to achieve a deeper understanding. This is a subtle process. We must plant the issue in our mind and hold it there, restraining ourselves from attacking it with our intellect. We must next allow our entire being to work with it without interference. Not only do we sit with it during the formal concentration of mindfulness training, but also we hold it with us at all times: when we walk, eat, and sleep. With patience, when the proper period of fertilization has occurred, and, if we can resist analyzing it, sudden insights will arise that will provide us with the understanding we need. Previous understandings will drop away as we begin to experience the insight and wisdom essential for a healthy life.

For example, let us concentrate on the issue of anger. When we experience recurrent difficulty in resolving conflict in a relationship, we automatically find ourselves becoming defensive and angry (It is much easier and more convenient to blame others than it is to observe, concentrate on, and understand our own perceptions and responses.). When the conflict is sufficiently prolonged and intense it may result in feelings of betrayal and helplessness. This will likely lead to more blame and anger and a continuing downward cycle, which can only conclude itself destructively. I imagine this scenario is as familiar to many of the readers as it is to me.

When we attempt to use our intellect to sort through these issues, we rarely get much further. Usually we rerun the same old tapes, which never provide us with insight and most often result in self-serving justifications of our anger. If we can 1) patiently shift our focus and attend to, observe, and concentrate on our own feelings (It may require hours or perhaps a day or two before we move from the delight of projecting onto others what is invariably ours.), 2) avoid the tendency to refocus on the other, 3) resist the tendency of our intellect to analyze the situation, 4) plant within our mind the intention to understand the situation and our angry response, and 5) practice concentration, we will invariably penetrate through our surface reactions and understandings to a liberating deeper understanding. This will progress at its own pace, so be patient.

For example, we will likely discover that our anger is a result of hurt. Underneath the hurt is often sadness. The sadness results from the feeling that I am not understood, cared for, or attended to. Continued concentration will reveal how familiar these feelings are, how we have repeated this pattern many times in our lives, and how much we have suffered from anger. Perhaps we will remember earlier life experiences that have fed the intensity of our reaction to the current situation. We may recall the early sources of our anger: the actions of a non-acknowledging or abusive immature parent, teacher, or significant other. Very slowly we will discover that, although others may be dis-acknowledging or insensitive, we do not have to feel disacknowledged or rejected. We are not required to take on their problems. As I have heard said before "another person's opinions about me are no business of mine."

While doing this work, strong emotions may arise that are linked to early childhood woundings. At these moments, you can return to mindfulness and observe these emotions, in contrast to becoming en-meshed in them. Observe them closely in order to learn more about their deeper sources.

As a complement to the mindfulness work, you can also choose to allow yourself, for the purposes of grieving these inner hurts, to experi-ence more fully the anger, hurt, and sadness as it is happening in that moment. This is a subtle process by which you simultaneously experience and observe your feelings, in contrast to either observing them with detachment or becoming inextricably enmeshed in them. As humans we have been given this capacity to soften and let go of intense feelings by feeling the feelings and grieving our losses, a process, which like grieving the death of a loved one, occurs over a period of time. This may take minutes, hours, or days. At this point, it is important to observe mindfully how and what you grieved and acknowledge the truth of your early losses. If this is an overwhelming experience it must be done with a counselor rather than by yourself.

As we work further with this issue, by ourselves and, when appropriate, with the assistance of a counselor, and continue to observe how our minds work, we will be released from the anger in proportion to our growing insight and realize that, as adults, our peace and balance need never be disturbed by the actions of others. Ironically, we will also discover there is no one to be angry at. The unhealthy and inappropriate behavior of others is a statement only about them. It requires nothing more from us than compassion and benign indifference. Using this information, let us concentrate on three difficult and important issues that touch many of our lives.

POWERLESSNESS

When mind-talk is about powerlessness, it fills us with feelings, thoughts, and images of helplessness, hopelessness, and victimization. As a result, we feel incompetent and inadequate. Unable to change our lives, we feel stuck and trapped and condemn ourselves to mental and physiologic distress. It is important to recognize that powerlessness is not preordained by our genes. Rather, it is acquired through our childhood experiences with authority, usually parental, and often confirmed in our experience as adults.

How does this happen? When Steve first came to my office, he complained about a persistent mild depression. He was in a job he disliked and found minimal satisfaction in his marriage. I saw him several times over the next twelve months. Despite his efforts, which included changes he initiated at work, discussions with his wife, relevant readings, and a seminar on goal setting, he remained depressed, and his life was essentially unchanged. As we discussed this further, it became evident that this intelligent, creative, and seemingly capable individual was helpless, powerless, and totally immobilized in his efforts to create change in his life. He acknowledged this and expanded upon it by verbalizing his confusion, frustration, and despair.

Steve learned powerlessness at home. There was only one way to do things in his home—his father's way. Confronted as a child with his father's insensitive use of authority, Steve was not allowed to express his opinions, negotiate his needs, or experience any sense of personal autonomy. His mother, who learned to live with her husband in quiet despair by resigning herself to a passive role, served as a model for Steve. With no alternatives, Steve learned to protect himself from the inappropriate use of parental authority by withdrawing, denying his needs, and resigning himself to powerlessness and helplessness in the only way he knew—his mother's way.

Learned powerlessness and helplessness not only result in mental distress, but also, as we discussed, they are transformed into physiologic stress. Attempting to demonstrate this, Steven Maier and Mark Laudenslager, noted researchers in PNI, conducted a series of experiments in which they documented the effects of learned helplessness and powerlessness on the immune system. [1] In an experiment, they gave one group of rats an inescapable series of tailshocks and another group escapable shocks; that is, the first group was restrained from escape, the second group was not. The surprising, but as yet tentative result, was that, when the restrained rats were tested, their immune systems showed suppression. The researchers concluded that the immune suppression was directly related to the helplessness the restrained rats experienced. This, and related research, is an early scientific confirmation that helplessness and powerlessness, learned early in life, reflect themselves in a high susceptibility to mental distress, physiologic stress, and their long-term consequences: acute and chronic illness.

As an adult, Steve's mind continues to talk powerlessness. Although he now has choices, his behavior continues to reflect this childhood attitude. Unfortunately, what saves the child often kills the adult. Steve now has only three alternatives: 1) to resign himself to feelings of powerlessness and helplessness, thus limiting the possibilities in his life, 2) to imitate his father's use of power; the power that comes from position and authority, the power to control and dominate, or 3) to see beyond his early childhood learnings to a potentially new and different source of power.

A Different Type of Power

Consider an alternate scenario. From infancy onward, one is respected and acknowledged. One's opinion is solicited and fully heard on all important issues. In school, one is judged in relationship to one's own potential rather than in comparison to others. One's teachers seek to understand and acknowledge one's unique gifts, encouraging their development. When it is time to choose a vocation, knowledgeable about one's special gifts, one chooses a path that will encourage an unfolding of one's individuality.

Such an individual learns a very different lesson from one who is thwarted. He or she develops an inner feeling of competence, confidence, and adequacy and learns about a different type of power: inner power. This form of power is natural, firm, sensitive, energizing, quiet, and permanent. It arises from a mind free of the restlessness and pervasive negative mind-talk of one who knows the fears and anxieties of growing up powerless. For this individual, authority is not an antidote to powerlessness but a natural expression of compassionate and wise leadership.

Inner power is a feeling we glimpse each time we accomplish a difficult task; achieve a sense of mastery in an athletic, vocational, or artistic endeavor; or, through the eyes of our loved one, feel the strength and adequacy that has always been ours. Our glimpse of this power becomes fleeting when we mistakenly believe the accomplishment, success, or lover to be the source of it. When the glow of achievement fades or our lover is gone, our power also appears to be gone. We did not understand the nature of inner power and the mind-talk that tells us that feelings of power come from outside sources. More mindfulness is necessary.

The first time I met Mary, she entered my office tearful and distraught, complaining about recurrent headaches and physical exhaustion. Married ten years, she stated with much distress that she could no longer tolerate being "trashed" anymore, that is, being verbally and emotionally abused. However, even though she was intelligent and creative, she could not imagine being unmarried and caring for herself.

She was immobilized in her attempts to leave a damaging relationship. During the interview, Mary acknowledged feelings of powerlessness and helplessness dating back to her childhood. I concluded the interview by asking her to ponder her alternatives: to learn to say no (the first step in moving beyond powerlessness) or to choose emotional death.

On her second visit Mary "bounced" into my office.

"I feel better," she stated. "I told him I was in therapy, I would no longer tolerate his abuse, and if it continued, I would move out."

Mary was feeling her power. I asked her to close her eyes and experience the power, creating an image of it in her mind.

"It feels like a steel plate in my chest. It feels strong but very hard and uncomfortable." I then asked her to concentrate and focus on the steel plate. Her attention to the steel plate would allow her to feel this sense of inner power (Any object or inner feeling can be used as a focal point to begin the movement into mindfulness.). If she could hold the focus, she would move into deeper aspects of mindfulness: contemplation and meditation. At that level she could begin to feel and understand the difference between a "forced" defensive power that results from fear and anger and is a desperate attempt at self-survival and a more natural inner power. Waiting a few minutes, I asked, "What is happening now?

"The plate is getting smaller, and I am feeling calmer and more peaceful."

Over the next five minutes, I carefully watched her breathing, the coloring of her skin, and the tenseness of her muscles, each an indication of her mental activity. As I observed her movement from attention to contemplation and into meditation, I asked her to make the steel plate disappear.

Several moments later she stated, "It's gone now."

"How do you feel?"

"Quieter, more relaxed, more peaceful."

"What happened to the power you were feeling, the power of the steel plate? Is it gone?"

"No! It's stronger, softer. I no longer have the discomfort in my abdomen. It feels more comfortable and natural to me. I feel I can do what I need to do in a quieter way."

I then asked her to go further into this feeling, the meditative state, and experience the vastness and strength of inner power. I warned her that initially it would be difficult to hold this power because mind-talk was still her predominant mental activity, and it would draw her back to powerlessness, rage, and further attempts at forced power. This brief glimpse at the peace and strength of inner power would, however, serve as her guide for the future.

While her eyes were still closed I further explained that, at times, those of us who have never known power must first experience it by forcing ourselves to say "no," create boundaries, and defend ourselves from people and situations that are harmful and unhealthy. When we get power in this way, we then must go within and learn the inner power that is stronger, compassionate, sensitive, does not deplete energy, and is permanent. This power does not come from hurt and rage, is not vulnerable to the opinions and actions of others, and is always present when we are in inner balance. She opened her eyes, and we concluded the hour-long visit.

Mary's first experience of her power was a result of her despair, fear, and rage. It was a beginning. If she can avoid becoming intoxicated with her newly discovered power (This type of power can be recognized by its punitive, controlling, and manipulative nature and is best handled by concentrating on and observing it.), a stage at which many become stuck for a lifetime, she will be able to move into a deeper and more sustaining inner power. She will also discover that authentic and sustaining power does not come from position, prestige, or gender. It comes from within. No one can take it from us. Only we can give it away by denying it, fearing it, or feeling guilty about it. Inner power is not used to control others, it is used to understand them. It is not used to manipulate but to serve. It does not separate individuals but connects them. It is not paraded around for all to see. It does its work gently and quietly.

EXERCISE 14:

DISCOVERING INNER POWER

Daily practice of the mindfulness training exercise (Exercise 3 in chapter 3), is essential for 1) training the mind in self-observation and 2) facilitating the meditative experience that silences mind-talk and promotes feelings of confidence and competence that are naturally present in the quiet mind.

The following exercise, which is not designed to be practiced daily, will assist you in understanding and integrating the information presented in the preceding section on powerlessness. Record the exercise on an audiotape allowing forty five minutes for its completion.

Comfortably seated, close your eyes and begin ten cycles of a complete breath. (pause two minutes) Follow the breathing with ten minutes of attention to your breath, fixing your attention on the rising and falling with inhalation and exhalation of your chest or abdomen or the sensation of air moving in and out of your nostrils (pause ten minutes)

Bring to awareness a past or current experience in which you felt a sense of power, control, and confidence. For some, it is difficult to recollect a time such as this. If it is difficult, create an imaginary experience and bring it to your awareness. In either case relive the experience as vividly as possible: Feel the feelings, see the sights, smell the smells, and think the thoughts. Enter into this experience as fully as you can. (pause five minutes)

Focus on the feelings of power, control, confidence, ease, and relaxation that were part of that moment. Notice where you feel the strength and power in your body. (pause one minute) What is the feeling like: warmth, tingling, vibrations? Whatever this feeling, intensify it and focus it into your solar plexus. Allow it to expand like a balloon being filled or to grow in strength like a powerful light or fire. For the next few minutes, work with intensifying and exaggerating this feeling. (pause three minutes)

When it can no longer be contained in this area of your body, allow the energy to move to your heart. Feel how your heart feels when it is filled with power. Continue to increase its intensity, slowly moving it throughout your body. (pause five minutes)

If there is a place in your body that feels unhealthy, direct the power to that space. Observe it filling the unhealthy area and note any changes. (pause three minutes)

Return now to the feeling of inner power. Notice how centered you feel and how little you need from the outside world. If the initial image is still present, let it go, while holding on to the feeling of confidence, competence, autonomy, and health. The image was necessary to assist in returning to the inner feeling of power: a feeling that is always available. With disciplined practice it can become an ordinary part of daily life. Continue to experience this feeling. (pause three minutes)

Bring to awareness a problem of current concern. (pause two minutes) Be sure not to get absorbed with mind-talk about this problem; just watch it from a position of inner strength. Who has the power, you or the problem? (pause one minute) Create two images: one of yourself and another as the problem. Which is bigger and looks more powerful? (pause two minutes)

Notice how tension develops if the problem begins to take over. You may feel your inner power dissipating. Do you wish to hold your power or give it to your problems or to other people? (pause one minute) Each time you begin to feel powerless, you give your power away. Stay with and intensify your inner power. Surrender your efforts at resolving the problem. Simply observe the problem without comment, maintaining your mindfulness. If you are distracted by mind-talk about the problem or other issues, return to your focus on the breath. (pause one minute)

When mindful, notice how issues diminish in intensity and power, easily lending themselves to resolution. Become aware of how centered and intact you feel. Notice the absence of fear. (pause one minute) Nothing has changed in the outer world, neither control nor manipulation were necessary; only self-change.

Slowly return to a focus on rising falling. Continue this for ten minutes. (pause ten minutes) Open your eyes, return to the time and space of the room, and review what you have learned in this exercise.

Very few of us have escaped the tendencies of our families and cultures to teach us helplessness and powerlessness. For some of us, this is a major and disabling problem, for others it is less so. In either case, it is often well hidden from view and wrapped in false outer power. This exercise is designed to demonstrate that each of us has within ourselves a reservoir of personal power. We were born into it, and those who tell you otherwise are violating you. Powerlessness is acquired and obscures a truthful view of our essential natures. When you feel powerless, use what you have learned to quiet your mind, remember your deeper and more essential self and observe what is happening. Work with breathing techniques, mindfulness, solitude, exercise, self-observation, and, most important, be patient, persistent, and remember your power through imagery, using its extraordinary capacity to assist you in reclaiming who you are.

EXERCISE 15:

GRIEVING OUR LOSSES

During the previous exercise, you may have become aware of feelings of powerlessness and victimization that were previously unknown to you or of greater intensity than previously recognized. If this occurs, you may set aside time to reexperience and grieve these feelings. Although this exercise follows our discussion of powerlessness, it can be used to work with any particularly strong emotions when they arise (this specifically applies to Exercises 16, 17, and 18). For some of us, the experience of helplessness and powerlessness can be overwhelming, *if you suspect this may be, do not attempt these exercises without a trained counselor.* Allow yourself a minimum of thirty minutes. Begin with ten minutes of a quieting exercise (the mindfulness training exercise or a breathing exercise).

When you have completed the ten minutes of quieting, bring to your mind a particular circumstance that recalls for you the feeling of powerlessness or victimization. To assist this process, allow yourself to return to this circumstance as fully as possible, noticing the particular place and people, seeing the sights, feeling the feelings, smelling the smells, and experiencing the physical sensations. Allow that feeling to intensify and move throughout your mind and body and observe how you feel when this feeling is present. (pause five minutes)
Continue by going backwards through your life recalling situations that were associated with these feelings. Observe them carefully, identify what these situations were, who was

present, how you responded and reacted. Go back as far as possible to the earliest moments in your life. (pause ten minutes) What does your mind feel like? What does your body feel like? (pause two minutes) Become aware of the patterns that connect these many experiences. See if you can identify the early sources of these *learned* feelings. Notice how pervasive these feelings have been in your life and how these feelings have structured your relationships and life experiences. (pause ten minutes)

If you begin to feel feelings of anger, sadness, and hurt, stay with them and allow the grieving process to take place. You will likely find the sequence of feelings to be anger, the desire to withdraw or attack, hurt, pain, and, finally, sadness. Allow these feelings to stay with you and observe how you relate to them, at all times allowing the feelings to follow their course (allow as long as necessary). *If this experience is overwhelming do not continue without a counselor.*

You will notice as you move through these feelings that you develop new insights and understandings. If you can stay with these feelings your mind and body, following the sadness, will always, in time, return to an inner peace and quiet. You will feel centered, and released from the distress. The ability of the mind and body to move through intense feelings to a peaceful state is in sharp contrast to what happens when we block feelings and permanently build in tension and anxiety into our lives. When you reach a peaceful state, observe how your body feels and be aware of how you can successfully move through, grieve, and learn from your feelings rather than "stuff" them (Allow whatever time you need for your observations.). When you are ready open your eyes and slowly reorient yourself to the room. Repeat this exercise whenever necessary, and remember to observe and follow your feelings whenever it is possible. It is essential to learn from your feelings rather than blocking them out, projecting them onto others, or acting them out.

It is very important to develop the capacity to "contain" your feelings. If you cannot sit and stay with your feelings, you will invariably, without thinking, "stuff" them or act them out, in either case causing yourself and others disease. The capacity to "contain" feelings, not suppress them but observe and experience them, will enable you to learn about them, discover their sources, and eventually diminish their impact on your life.

LONELINESS

In the study of human relationships, considerable research links death of a spouse, poor marital quality, marital disruption (separation or divorce), and a single person's life-style to stress and disease. The link between loneliness, loss, stress, depression, and illness is slowly emerging. Understanding the dynamics of loneliness and the related issues of love and relationship can help to move us beyond a common form of mental and physiologic distress to a healthier and more life-sustaining approach to these important and difficult human experiences.

As human beings we seem to need each other. Loving oneself and others is not a luxury in life: it is a necessity for healthy living. Community, the sharing and interaction with others, whether it be one or one hundred, facilitates our growth and development. Love gives us hope and an opportunity to feel ourselves as whole. Yet, as the psychologist Erich Fromm, speaking of relationships, has stated in his book, *The Art of Loving*, "There is hardly any activity, any enterprise, which is started with such tremendous hopes and expectations, and yet, which fails so regularly, as love." There is much loneliness in our society. It is neither related nor limited to living without an intimate mate. It exists in many marriages and "stable" relationships.

Loneliness is an attitude, a mental perspective that associates being alone with feelings of sadness and emptiness accompanied by a strong longing for another. Only when the special other is found and reciprocates our longing does loneliness seem to cease. Three basic misperceptions form the basis for this attitude: 1) love is something that comes to us from the outside, that is, finding the right person to love us, 2) love is found and secured through relationship, and 3) love and relationship are one and the same. Each of these misperceptions, acquired early in life and frequently reaffirmed through our adult experiences, is the source of much of the suffering and distress associated with relationships.

It is important to understand that it is not the fact of being alone that results in emotional and physical distress. Loneliness results from a lack of being present with ourselves. We are so busy looking for the right person or complaining that the one we have does not understand our "needs" and "style," that we rarely look within to question what we are looking for or why we do not find it. There is a difference between the healthy desire to share the intimacy and companionship of another and the unhealthy search for relationship as an *antidote* to the anxiety and pain of loneliness. The latter can only be resolved by first developing a healthy relationship with oneself.

It took many years, great effort, and much pain to discover this truth in my own life. After years of difficult and troubling relationships, I was finally forced by desperation and an irrepressible need to understand what had gone wrong, a need motivated by a commitment not to relive such an experience; to move beyond surface explanations to a deeper comprehension of my role in these relationships. I was convinced that I could not move on until I understood it. What I was to discover taught me much about loneliness, the effect on my adult life of my early childhood experiences, and my capacity to move beyond these experiences to a sustained experience of love.

After attempting for many months to sort through this problem, to my surprise, while traveling by air from one city to another, the first important clue suddenly, without expectation, appeared. A long-ago image reentered my awareness; the stored memory of an event that occurred twenty years previously. It was the image of a face. Years ago, while visiting the Uffizi Gallery in Florence, Italy, my attention unexpectedly became riveted on the face of Venus in Botticelli's renowned painting, *The Birth of Venus.* Focused on what I perceived to be the warmth, gentleness, and serenity of this face, much to my surprise, feelings, with an intensity previously unknown to me, began to arise and fill my heart: feelings of openness, softness, peacefulness, and love. I lingered for a considerable period of time, delighted, intrigued, and transfixed with these new feelings.

Suddenly, similar to the feeling that comes when the last few pieces of a jigsaw puzzle rapidly move into place, I began to recognize how I had sought to transfer the Venus face and the feelings associated with it to the face of very real women. I had spent many years looking for the "right" woman who could again unlock the feelings that I first experienced that morning at the Uffizi. I was seeking the special person, the special relationship with which to feel my love. When I finally imagined I had "found her," it was not long until I was faced with the suffering that comes when one misunderstands the truth and becomes dependent and attached to another for that which can only be provided by one's self. I slowly, and, at first, tentatively, began to understand that the love I was feeling within had more to do with me than with a painting or another person.

Intellectual understanding is an important first step in "getting it inside." Understanding at a deeper level is, however, essential to free oneself from the strong pull of misperceived ideas. This occurred several years later, when, through the unconditional loving gifts of another, I was able to directly, convincingly, and permanently experience and finally own the power, presence, and depth of my love. Through her active support and love, and my readiness, I finally understood that love had always been within me. Though previously activated by others, I finally discovered that it belonged to me. I could experience it any time I wanted to. I merely had to drop my unneeded defenses, push away the heavy veils, open my heart, and love would be there. In this "flash" of a moment the work of years was culminated as I accepted the power, capacity, and fullness of love.

I discovered that what I had experienced in the empty face of Botticelli's Venus (a face available to accept anything placed on it) was the projection of my own love and my own feminine qualities, qualities that had long been hidden from my view. The intervening years were years of necessary preparation that would allow me to finally reclaim and "own" what had always been mine.

This brief, transforming relationship was completed in a few weeks. Yet, the recognition that love is eternally present within me and unrelated to the presence of another was an essential step that replaced illusion with truth. Although the old misperceptions sneak back every once in a while, they are quickly recognized and thus deemed powerless. I no longer believe it is possible to *receive* love from relationship or another person, but rather that others offer the opportunity to share the love that is already present.

Although intimate relationships are always filled with the complexity of two different individuals learning to understand and accept the differences of another, I discovered they can be free of suffering. They are no longer the central driving force of my life. With energy freed from my previous misconceived pursuit of love, I can now enjoy love and relationship and use my energy for other important creative tasks of life. The journey from the first tentative feelings of inner love awakened by the Botticelli Venus to the ownership and full experience of love spanned a period of twenty years.

Not everyone seeks to fill an inner emptiness through relationship. There are many ways to try to fill a heart that has not met and owned its capacity for love. These misplaced efforts include the desire for material possessions, power, fame, and drugs. In a sense they are all drugs.

A Different Kind of Love

I discovered that love does not reside outside but, rather, within. Lovers show us the love that is given naturally to each of us; they are not the source of our love. They cannot take our love from us, any more than they can give it to us. They are only mirrors. Only we can disen-franchise ourselves from our love, by not opening to what has always been within us. When we narrow love down to another person we cheat ourselves of the healing possibility that is at all times available to each of us.

There is no hierarchy in love, no better or worse love, no more or less love. There are no conditions in love. There is no need to seek love, since it is already present within you awaiting you to "remember" it. We can all discover the astonishing truth that it is possible to love a person, a tree, or an automobile in exactly the same way. All that differs is the form of the relationship. You live with a person, sit under a tree, and drive an automobile. In each case, the love is the same. The quiet mind of meditation, freed from the narrow cultural perspectives on love, can directly experience its omnipresence. There is enough love for everyone: There is no need for loneliness.

Love, relationship, and sex are three separate experiences that can, at times, be joined in an intimate relationship. Love comes from within, it is personal and spiritual. It may or may not be shared in a relationship. Relationship is an interactive experience between two individuals, drawn together by a mutual attraction, in which both individuals share their individual love, life experiences, and goals for the future. Sex is the physical joining of individuals. It may or may not be part of a relationship or part of a shared love experience.

For those who have not experienced and taken possession of their own love, no further words can help but to offer assurance that it is there. With continued contemplation of this issue and practice of the mindfulness training exercise, you will, in time, create a caring relationship with yourself and, in the peace and quiet of the meditative state, learn to experience your own love. When you are finally in a state of love, you will no longer need to seek love because it will be everywhere.

THE SKILLS OF RELATIONSHIP

Relationships teach us about our own love, which we often see for the first time in the receptive eyes of our beloved. Relationships also nurture and heal. Although love is a natural experience, it is not enough for relationship. We need to learn specific skills for relationship, skills that we are not born with and seldom learn in school or from our friends. We learn these skills by maintaining a high level of mindfulness, practicing open communication, and, when necessary, seeking the guidance of knowledgeable people or resources.

Healthy relationships diminish our susceptibility to stress and enhance our capacity for a healthy mind-style and life-style. The result is less stress and more relaxation. This mental state or attitude, in addition to providing more moments of satisfaction and joy, becomes transformed through the chemical messengers of the brain into a healthy physiologic balance.

Several key issues are sources of recurrent distress in many relationships. You can test whether they are stress points for you by focusing on them when your mind is clear and quiet. If you discover that they are of current concern, quiet your mind-talk, and consider them at length.

No One Can Love Me More Than I Love Myself

As apparent as this may seem, few of us act as though this statement were true. Some of us demand love of others in proportion to our lack of love for ourselves. When we feel love for ourselves, we feel confident, alive, spontaneous, and joyful. Then, our heart is open, undefended, and available to receive and experience the love of another. When we feel disdain for ourselves and feel unlovable we build walls that separate us from others. Others, either frustrated that their love cannot be received through thick walls or fatigued from the energy it requires to love a person who does not love himself, give up and go away affirming and solidifying within us the illusion that we are unlovable. The health-promoting idea is not to seek love from others but to discover love within oneself. When the latter is accomplished, love is available wherever one sets one's eyes.

No One Can Give Me What I Cannot Give Myself

This concept complements the preceding concept. When we look to others as antidotes for our loneliness, powerlessness, feelings of deprivation, poor self-image, lack of achievement, or persistent anxiety, we become dependent on our loved ones to give us what ultimately we must give ourselves. Dependency on another for what we can provide for ourselves usually brings disaster. Sooner or later we will not get what we imagine we need, and anger and resentment enter the previously pristine relationship. Healthy relationships compel us, often with great pain, to return inside and work with our imagined inadequacies until we can discover the love within us. Often, the great gift in a relationship is not that it gives us what we want, but that it denies us what we want.

Giving Is Not About Getting

Giving is frequently the most controlling and manipulative action in relationships. To give freely is to give without any expectation, stated or unstated, of anything in return. Giving has nothing to do with reciprocity or fairness. Reciprocity and fairness are about business transactions, not loving relationships. If you do not get what you feel you need in a relationship, deal with that directly—not by *asking* and *demanding* disguised as *giving*, but by discussing your legitimate needs. Giving must be a clean and pure action, which is its own reward. Each time you give, be sure you have attached no strings. Then, you will not end up with health-threatening resentment and anger, and the other will not end up guilty over a presumed obligation that may not or cannot be fulfilled.

Difference Is Not Rejection

The most difficult aspect of any relationship is recognizing and accepting that the other person is different from me. I would like to repeat this statement for emphasis. *The most difficult aspect of any relationship is recognizing and accepting that the other person is different from me.* An introvert, who becomes quiet and gets pensive when faced with anxiety, is not rejecting the extravert who wants to talk—he is self-reflecting. This is how the introvert works with anxiety. The extravert, who is endlessly verbal when anxious, is not attacking the introvert who needs to be quiet and self-reflective—he is dealing with anxiety in the only way he knows, talking. When one individual in the relationship needs more space and time alone than the other, this is not rejection, but the difference between two people's needs.

Honoring difference may at times mean that it is not possible for two individuals to maintain their love in the form of an intimate relationship, or it may mean that each can expand his style and learn from the other. Love is not enough for an intimate relationship: shared interests and reasonably compatible styles are necessary for successful intimate relationships. To deal with the conflict that arises as we attempt to change another person, we must go inside ourselves and honestly examine our needs, personal style, and manner of relating to the other person's differences. We may find, with new perspectives, a new appreciation for the diversity of personalities that we experience in all our relationships each day.

Separateness Is Not Withdrawal

As with dancing, the skill of moving from union to separateness, and from separateness to union, is a finely tuned, intuitive, and rhythmic act. Next to seeing and acknowledging the differences in individuals, it is perhaps the second most difficult aspect of relationship. We must learn to remain both separate and together and must be able to do both at precisely the same moment. Too frequently, we lose our individuality in relationship and with it aspects of our personality, interests, and talents that are covered over and forgotten as we become absorbed into the other. The alternative is defensively to maintain our separateness for fear of losing ourselves. In either case, a healthy relationship is not possible, and the effort required to maintain either alternative can create stressful conditions that affect health. Relationship paradoxically requires both union and separateness.

Only I Need To Change

Your responsibility in a relationship is always to look within and ask the questions: "How have I created this problem?," "Why am I reacting this way?," and "How can I change?" To understand how, start with yourself. If you can change in a way that enables you to give more freely, to better respect and accept the difference in individual styles, to learn to care for and assert your important needs, and to express your feelings and these needs *directly*, the result will be a healthier relationship with whomever you are. The other individual, if he/she chooses, is free to ask or not ask the same questions.

I Am Never Alone

Do not confuse loneliness and aloneness. Aloneness can be restorative, a sought-after state that is essential for self-growth and spirituality. Loneliness is usually dreaded. A relationship can never be an antidote for loneliness. If it is seen in this way, it is likely that you will ultimately feel alone even in the presence of the other person. The antidote to loneliness begins with mindfulness and increasingly regular experience of the deeper self that is always present and available. This experience of connection with ourselves can teach us connection with others and the natural world in a fearless, unchanging, and invulnerable manner. This capacity to experience the deeper self is the foundation upon which a relationship with another can be developed most successfully.

It is important to restate that loneliness is a distressful inner state resulting from misperceptions about love and relationship. Love and relationship are different experiences. Not to know this is to confuse the two, making it more difficult to accomplish either. *Love* is a formless, permanent, unconditional experience, a feeling that comes from the heart and does not require an object, person or thing. The experience of unconditional love is a capacity of the deeper self, the self of mindfulness. *Relationship* is form. It describes a conditional and often impermanent way that we choose to interact with each other. It very much involves our personality with its wants, needs, hopes, and dreams. Love may or may not be a part of the relationship. The relationship may last for days or for decades. You may lose a relationship, but you never need to lose the experience of love. Mindfulness helps us in recognizing our misperceptions, and discovering the important truths about love and relationship.

QUICK RECAP

- There is a direct relationship between loneliness and disease. Research suggests that loneliness can result in an increased susceptibility to stress and depression, which is reflected in physiologic changes that increase the risk of disease.
- Loneliness is an attitude based on three misperceptions: a) love is found outside of us, b) relationship is the source of love, and c) love and relationship are one and the same.

EXERCISE 16:

MINDFUL RELATIONSHIPS

Record the following exercise on an audiotape. Observe the pauses and allow one hour.

Comfortably seated, close your eyes, and bring to your attention the image and awareness of an individual with whom you have or have had unresolved issues. Allow your mind to talk freely about this relationship. Listen to its concerns, resentment, anger, and to the many conversations it has had or will have about your relationship with this person.

It is likely that your mind has seen the issues in this relationship in a protective and defensive manner. This is how mind-talk often expresses itself. It relives the same thoughts, rarely providing new insights or creative alternatives that can assist in healing disordered relationships. Continue observing your mind-talk for an additional five minutes. (pause five minutes)

Next, move this image from your awareness and enter mindfulness by bringing your attention to the breath, as you have done in the mindfulness training exercise. Notice how difficult it is to shift to mindfulness when your mind-talk has focused on negative thoughts. Allow yourself ten minutes, or whatever time is needed, to enter the mindful state. You will know when you are there by recognizing the quiet mind and body, and the feelings of peacefulness, harmony, balance, inner strength, and spaciousness. Notice how defensiveness and protectiveness are gone. The mindful self feels secure, abundant, and invulnerable. (pause ten minutes)

Remaining at all times centered in your mindful self, bring to awareness the image and sense of the person you worked with in the previous exercise. Remain present but removed and detached from this individual, as if he/she were a neutral object. Focus your attention on the image or sense of this person. If mind-talk begins, clear your mind by refocusing on the image as if it were the "rising-falling" of your training exercise.

As you remain focused on this individual and without mind-talk, you will begin to notice other aspects of this person. Underlying his/her behavior you may notice fear, hurt, anxiety, and pain. You may be able to see back to the layers of his/her earlier life and the distress and suffering that has led him/her to this point in life. You may become aware of the purpose that has brought both of you together and the learning that is to come from this relationship.

Continue to focus and allow the mindful self to take you beyond these issues to a deeper awareness of this individual. If you remain in mindfulness, you will begin to experience this individual at deeper levels that can free your relationship from its current perspectives and boundaries. You may appreciate this individual's way of being—his/her similarities and differences. You may understand that we all take different paths to the same place and that, what may seem odd and peculiar in the path of another, is merely another person's unique way of finding love and joy. However disturbed it may appear, this way is the best that he or she can do at the present moment.

You may recognize that, although you may not be able to share a relationship with this person or your relationship may be quite limited, you are able to share love. You may choose to hold this love silently or share it verbally. Love does not require the participation of the other. As you feel and experience love, notice how it is contained within you and does not require the other person for its existence. Notice how, inside your body, you feel a sense of aliveness, warmth, wholeness, and harmony.

You are now free to know that love is inside you and requires nothing and no one. It only requires opening your nondefended heart. Hold this feeling while you move away from the awareness and the image of the other individual and remain with this feeling for an additional ten minutes. (pause ten minutes)

Open your eyes and fix your attention on an object in front of you. Notice how this object feels to you when you are open and loving. Become aware of the connection with this object, its warmth, beauty, and its aliveness and expression of the unity, flow, energy, and love that constitutes life.

Get up from your seat and move around. Perhaps go outdoors. Remain in the mindful and loving state as you experience individuals and nature. Walk slowly, with full awareness of your body, mind, and the outside world. Stop for a few moments and focus on one particular object. Notice how much it can teach you about life. The longer you linger the more you can learn, the more it will become alive for you, and the more you can experience the unity and connection of all things.

This exercise does not need to end in one hour. It can continue for the remainder of your life. It is more likely, however, that the pulls of daily life will draw you from your participation in this new way of looking at life into the world of mind-talk. This is as it should be. We must learn to move between both worlds—inner and outer. With training and practice in mindfulness, you will be able to at all times direct your mind, locating your attention where you wish it to be.

Intimate relationships force us to see everything about ourselves that we never wanted to see. This is their gift and their pain. If you can "use" relationship, it can become a powerful vehicle through which you can discover who and what you are. If you avoid what relationships can teach you, by blaming the other (others obviously also have their own problems), looking for the "right" person, withdrawing, or numbing your pain with possessions, drugs, or false power you will lose yourself and the beauty and brilliance of a healthy intimate relationship.

It is important to remember that healthy supportive relationships not only result in joy and peace, but also have a clear impact on physiologic health. I have reviewed the research that supports this conclusion in earlier chapters. For reemphasis, I will restate the findings of this research: 1) loss of a loved one invariably results in increased levels of ill-health, and unexpected death in the surviving spouse, 2) marital disharmony is related to ill-health, 3) recently separated couples have an increased incidence of ill-health, 4) divorce is one of the most stressful and disease-inducing life events, and 5) loneliness increases susceptibility to stress and its related disorders.

To the extent that we can master the capacity for such relationships, we can tap into the healing power that comes from the emotional and physical "healing touch" of others, as well as that of our own love. There are few who would doubt its healing potency, and there are no toxic side effects. Healthy relationship is not a luxury.

DEPRIVATION

We feel deprived when our perceived needs are unmet—when we feel that someone or something is unable to provide for our needs. When we project this feeling on the outside world we see it as a world of scarcity. For some of us, deprivation and scarcity is a way of life, there is never enough security, money, time, or love. Life becomes an endless struggle with the outside world: a struggle to meet our needs and reduce the anxiety of the mind that fears deprivation. When the mind finally quiets, and our needs appear met, another fear, the fear of losing what we have attained, asserts its control and continues the unceasing anxiety and struggle that is characteristic of the mentality of deprivation and scarcity.

To live with the feeling of never having enough is to be always searching for the money, power, position, possessions, or lovers that will finally relieve the anxious and frantic search. We accumulate more and more, and, to our dismay, still need more and more. Whenever we are still, we start moving. It is as if when we stop, we are falling behind in our race against the forces of scarcity and deprivation, a race that can never be won until we change directions.

When the mind talks deprivation and scarcity, it is replaying old messages. It talks as if we are living in a prehistoric era when each day was a struggle to find food, wild animals roamed freely, and human savagery was uncontrolled. It ignores today's replacements: supermarkets, zoos, and the rule of law. Few of us lack the basic physical needs of life. What we lack is love and respect for ourselves, trust in the abundance of the world and of our being, a faith in the capacity of the life process to provide us with what we need, and the knowledge and wisdom that can shift us beyond the mind-talk of deprivation and scarcity to the deeper, achievable reality of abundance.

Thinking, feeling, imaging, and sensing deprivation inevitably leads an individual to disappointment, frustration, anxiety, and depression. The research in PNI and the clinical investigation of individuals with serious disease suggests that depression, like stress, powerlessness, and loneliness, suppresses the immune system and shifts the body physiology in a direction of increased susceptibility to disease. Like the antidote for powerlessness and loneliness, the antidote for a mentality of deprivation is a shift in perspective, one that requires an inward turn.

ABUNDANCE

Deep within our mind, each of us has some feeling, memory, or image of feeling healthy and fully alive. These feelings of abundance, although they may be rare for those struggling with unhappiness, financial problems, or the endless demands of daily life, are satisfying. They can bring feelings of peace and completeness. In these moments, we may even experience ourselves as fully healthy. Abundance and wholeness, although too often forgotten, are always awaiting our return home.

There was a time when meadow, grove, and stream,
To earth, and every common sight,
> *To me did seem*
> *Apparelled in celestial light,*
The glory and freshness of a dream.
It is not now as it has been of yore—
> *Turn whereso'er I may,*
> *By night or day,*
The things which I have seen I now can see no more.

WILLIAM WORDSWORTH,
Ode: Intimations of Immortality

Our remembrance of wholeness and delight, often experienced in the early blush of a new relationship, the quiet of meditation, the joy of a walk in the woods, or, for too many, in the brief surge of a mind-altering drug, is both our possibility and our pain. The possibility is, in Wordsworth's words, the recovery of "the hour of the splendour in the grass, of the glory of the flower. . . ." Our pain is that we only have brief glimpses and remembrances of these feelings and are unaware of the knowledge necessary to return to them.

Replacing this loss of long ago, we have instead a path, a direction, and an operator's manual, products of our family and culture, which we are told will provide us with health and happiness. After years of climbing the prescribed ladders and perhaps even reaching the top, it is painful to discover we have achieved little of the peace, joy, and happiness we were promised. We feel cheated in two ways, 1) we followed the rules and ended up empty-handed, and 2) we do not have the resources to get what we need.

As I have stated earlier in this chapter, we each have the means to discover and bring to our lives all that we need. We can have abundance, just as we can have personal power and meaningful relationships, in proportion to our capacity to live with a quiet and mindful mind. The mindful self knows that abundance is not about getting, but giving; not about having, but letting go; not about a depriving world but an ignored inner self.

Collecting people, possessions, and power provides only a moment of peace or satisfaction in an otherwise frantic life. On the other hand, letting go of the expectation that the acquisition of people and things is the only source of satisfaction opens a new possibility. To watch this possibility emerge, each day, in many ordinary individuals, convinces me of the ease with which we can all live with feelings of abundance.

The first step toward abundance is the simple, yet very difficult acknowledgment: I have failed to meet my healthy needs reasonably in a manner that consistently provides me with feelings of satisfaction and abundance. Unless you take this first step, you cannot make further progress. You must move beyond the illusion that you will achieve peace by manipulating the outside world. Accepting this piece of reality is difficult. It defies much, if not all, of what we have learned. It is not easy to let go of what we know for the uncertainty of the unknown. Breakdown must always precede breakthrough.

The second step is to recognize and acknowledge that abundance cannot be achieved in the outside world until we have achieved it in our inner world. This may appear to be a step backward. In truth, it is the first step in the right direction and a step over which we have control. It is forced upon us by the suffering and distress that comes from the repeated failure of a way of living that does not work. If this step seems inappropriate and premature, you will likely continue to live from the unhealthy attitude of deprivation and scarcity.

The third step is the daily, disciplined practice of mindfulness. With patient practice, as you reverse years of ineffective effort, you increasingly will experience inner abundance. This feeling will be characterized by a sense of spaciousness, expansiveness, calm, and, for many, the first adult experience of complete satisfaction with few, if any, needs or wants. This feeling can extend into your daily activities, even though it requires you to remain centered in mindfulness while carrying out your responsibilities.

As you increasingly experience abundance in your mind and body, a strange new feeling emerges. The outer world, previously seen as a place of scarcity, will begin to appear abundant in direct proportion to your inner feelings of abundance. Nothing has changed except your inner perspective. People and things that previously brought you grief can now enhance your feelings of abundance. Paradoxically, the very world you struggled with and sought to change through control, manipulation, and an unending compulsive drive for perfection in work and relationship has changed. The less you demand of it, the more it gives you.

QUICK RECAP

- We feel deprived when our perceived needs are unmet; when we feel that someone or something is unable to provide for our needs.
- When we project this feeling onto the outside world, we see it as a world of scarcity.
- The feeling of deprivation, like powerlessness and loneliness, is an acquired misperception of childhood.
- Current research in PNI suggests that loneliness, which frequently leads to stress and depression, alters the immune and other body systems in a way that increases susceptibility to disease.
- Through the practice of mindfulness, individuals recognize that abundance must, and can, be found in the inner world.

EXERCISE 17:

OBSERVING DEPRIVATION AND ABUNDANCE

Record this exercise on an audiotape allowing thirty minutes.

Sit comfortably in a chair or lie on your back and close your eyes. Allow your mind to wander over the events of the week. Follow the mind-talk and label each thought, image, and feeling as deprivation or abundance. Criticism, cynicism, anger, resentment, stress, and negative judgements are a few examples of perceived deprivation. (pause five minutes)

Continue to follow the mind-talk and label the thoughts, feelings, and images of abundance. Joy, delight, calm, satisfaction, and contentment are examples of perceived abundance. Count the number of mind-talk statements that reflect deprivation, and the number that reflect abundance. (pause five minutes)

With what color do you "color" the world when you are feeling deprived? Does it have a shade of gray? (pause one minute) Does the outer world feel scarce, hostile, and uncooperative? (pause one minute) Become aware of the interplay between your inner attitude and the perceived outer reality. (pause one minute)

Notice when your feelings are those of abundance. Now what color is the world? (pause one minute) Does it seem scarce or abundant? Do the outer world and other people become quiet, calm, and nonthreatening in proportion to your own feelings of abundance? (pause one minute) Notice how your mind tends to draw you from feelings of abundance back to feelings of fear and deprivation. (pause one minute)

Create a little movie theater. Sitting in the second row, watch a movie of one day in your life. Observe the moments of deprivation and abundance. What and who triggers these feelings? What is the effect of sleep, food, exercise, and friends? (pause five minutes)

Do you have any control over which perspective your mind is focused on, or do outer events and people have "mind control" over you? Notice how your mind-talk is constantly shifting and changing its perspective, often with a strong emphasis on deprivation. (pause two minutes)

Leave the little movie theater, open your eyes, and slowly return to the room. When resuming your regular daily activities, maintain an awareness of your attitude: abundance versus deprivation. What triggers feelings of abundance and of deprivation? How does your environment effect your attitudes and feelings? You will slowly discern the truth; that although deprivation can be real and the source of much suffering, for most of us who are fortunate to live in abundant societies, deprivation is in the mind and *not* in external circumstances.

EXERCISE 18:

REMEMBERING

Every infant is born abundant and whole. Next time you are around one, watch carefully. They are not yet limited by their soon-to-be-discovered teachers who, in most instances, have long ago lost their sense of wholeness and abundance. Because we are each born this way, we have within ourselves the remembrance of this feeling. The following exercise will assist you in remembering this feeling. As I have discovered in my practice and workshops, everyone can rediscover it, and, as expected, the descriptions are usually quite similar.

Record this exercise on an audiotape allowing thirty minutes.

Comfortably seated, close your eyes. Use the next five minutes to quiet your mind and body. (pause five minutes) Slowly "change channels" and enter mindfulness by focusing on the breath. Continue this for the next ten minutes. (pause ten minutes)

Next, bring to your awareness a time in your life in which you experienced the feelings of abundance. If you cannot recall such a time, make a mental note that this was not possible, and create an imaginary moment of delight, spontaneity, and well-being. (pause two minutes) Immerse yourself in this moment as if it were happening right now. See the sights, feel the feelings, hear the sounds. Notice the sun or wind against your skin, the temperature, the sense of being attuned to all that is happening. Continue this for the next five minutes. (pause five minutes)

Become aware of the feeling of abundance in your mind and body. Where do you feel this feeling? What is it like? (pause one minute) Is it in your stomach, your chest, or another part of your body? For the next several minutes, intensify and exaggerate this feeling until you are completely filled with it. (pause three minutes) What does your body feel like now? What does the room and outer world feel like? (pause two minutes) It is important to know, in your mind and body, the feeling of abundance. It can serve as a marker for health.

What are your thoughts and images? (pause two minutes) As with your feelings, note the inner experience of abundance. Notice how your thoughts and images are different. Notice how filled you feel and the relative lack of needs or wants. (pause two minutes) There is enough love, security, and joy for everyone because we each carry our own. Continue observing this

experience in your mind and body for the next ten minutes.
(pause ten minutes)

Slowly open your eyes and reorient yourself to the room.
Stand up, walk around, and experience delight in all the
wonders around you. Use the next ten minutes to experience
how different everything appears from the perspective of inner
abundance.

CONCLUSION

Each of these three important mind-body states, powerlessness, loneliness, and deprivation, appears to be directly related to the development
of distress and disease. They are all acquired as a result of retained
childhood misperceptions (Young children lack the life experience and
discriminative capacities to distinguish truth from the falsehood that is
too frequently passed on from parent to child.). Practicing conscious
living and applying mindfulness to the investigation of your unhealthy
psychologic mind-talk will inevitably free you from these misperceptions and provide the opportunity for inner power, connectedness, and
abundance.

I strongly suggest that you return to this chapter and its exercises at
regular intervals until you develop the capacity to watch your mind
carefully and precisely and investigate its mind-talk as part of your daily
routine. Deeply ingrained patterns take a long time to change. Just
when you think you have moved beyond them, they have a tendency to
reappear in new and disguised forms.

While we are learning these new practices it is important to recognize that we are not as yet Buddha or Jesus. If this were so, the mind of
anyone in our presence would rise to meet our level of illumination. As
it is unlikely that many of us will achieve full enlightenment in the next
few years, it is important, while practicing the path of mindfulness, to
be with those people and experiences that support your goal and be wise
enough to move away from people and things that, in your early stages
of training, pull you from your centeredness.

By training ourselves in mindfulness and self-regulation, we assume
control over our lives and fully develop these unique capacities that

define human existence. Mindfulness and self-regulation provide the opportunity for us to use (rather than be used by) the experiences of the past and present to self-invent the future. We take control of our own evolution: a powerful possibility requiring an equally powerful effort.

Chapter 8

WORKING THE PROGRAM

In preceding chapters, we considered a new approach to health, self-healing, which relies on our inner resources and capacities to help us to reclaim our possibilities and achieve peaceful and joyous lives of full health. We learned that mindfulness starts the healing process by assisting us in becoming more aware of our lives, enabling us to determine the truth of our lives, and then steering us away from unhealthy mind-talk toward healthy attitudes and healthy self-regulating actions. If we patiently persist in our efforts, mindfulness and self-regulation progressively will correct physical and emotional distress, reduce our susceptibility to disease, and promote a new way of living. Our experience of ourselves is enriched, and we are on our way to full healing.

In this chapter, we will put it all together and see how it works. Remember that a model is not real life. It is a blueprint and teaching guide; something from which to work and expand upon from your own experience. Figure 8.1 diagrams the process of mind-body healing that was discussed in previous chapters. This chapter will help you to understand how to move step-by-step through the healing program and how healing can become a way of life.

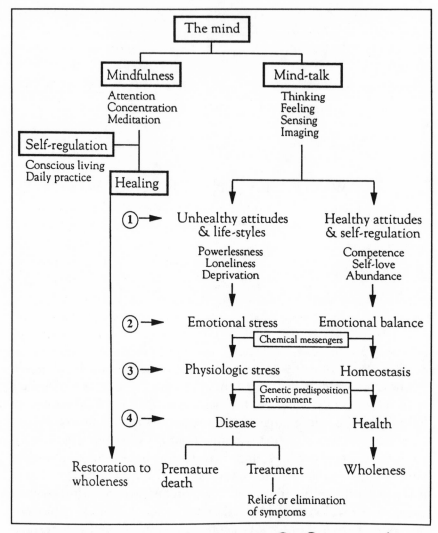

Figure 8-1. The process of mind-body healing. ①→④ are potential intervention points where a mind-body healing program can be initiated.

Beginning at the top of the figure, healing starts in the mind whenever we finally decide to take charge of and observe our lives. At birth we are filled with optimism, trust, resilience, and wholeness, but, as we grow and develop through our interaction with others, our minds collect an increasingly large file of memories, stored information, that stimulates the predominant activity of our mind, mind-talk. Although rarely experienced, our mind also contains the natural, and frequently undeveloped, capacity for mindfulness, attention, concentration, and meditation.

Mind-talk, expressed through the inner dialogue of thoughts, images, sensations, and feelings, results in a set of attitudes that guide our actions and basic life-styles. When our past experiences have left us with healthy attitudes (for example, competence, self-love, and abundance), our actions naturally create health. When our attitudes are unhealthy (for example, powerlessness, loneliness, and deprivation), our life-styles are invariably unhealthy.

We are all a mixture of healthy and unhealthy attitudes and actions. The former will move us down the far right side of the diagram toward emotional balance, homeostasis, and health; the latter will take us toward emotional stress, physiologic stress, and disease. Although there are times when we feel the predominance of our healthy side, and, thus better levels of health, we are inevitably pulled back toward the fear, worry, and anxiety that result from our unhealthy attitudes and actions. Full health and healing do not come in pieces and parts, it requires that *all* of our attitudes and actions be healthy. Lest the reader feel a bit overwhelmed by this thought, we must remember that this is a process, a direction, and a life intention, not a goal to be realized in thirty days without ups and downs, back and forths, and intermittent plateaus.

As discussed in preceding chapters and as is shown in Figure 8-1, unhealthy attitudes lead to both emotional and physiologic stress. Because we are so accustomed to living with daily stress, we may be unaware of its increasing presence in our lives. Nevertheless, a stressed mind activates the body's messengers systems (neuropeptide chemicals and the autonomic and central nervous systems) which move stress from the mind to the body. Most individuals are surprised by the "sudden" appearance of "physical" disease. This, unfortunately, is when individuals usually arrive at my office, complaining not of stress, but a physical ailment.

Disease usually results from the interaction of multiple predisposing factors. Figure 8-1 shows the most important of these factors: stress, genetic tendencies, and harmful environments. Together, they produce a pattern of illness that is unique for each individual. The usual immediate response is to seek treatment through the traditional medical model. This inclination may be appropriate and necessary. For many, treatment will, for a time, abort the disease by relieving or eliminating symptoms, which allows for the opportunity to initiate a healing program. Rarely, however, does a treatment approach result in a cure, and it does little to cure or alter the subtle source of disease, an unhealthy mind, leaving the individual at an increased risk for recurrent illness and, eventually, premature disability or death. For most individuals, this late outcome is preceded by years of a stressful, unhappy, and unsatisfied life.

Healing starts when we shift our attention from treatment to healing. As Figure 8-1 shows, this shift begins when we start to train our minds in attention, concentration, and meditation, the three aspects of mindfulness that help us "clean" our mind. Through daily practice of the mindfulness training process (see chapter 3, Exercise 3) we can master the skills of mindfulness and apply them (see chapters 5, 6, and 7) to reducing stress, changing unhealthy attitudes and life-styles, and promoting self-healing.

Figure 8-1 shows that, by using mindfulness and self-regulation, we can initiate healing at four possible intervention points: 1) harmful attitudes and life-styles, 2) emotional stress, 3) physiologic stress, and 4) overt disease. The longer we wait to intervene, for example, waiting until the appearance of the signs and symptoms of disease, the more effort is required and the more difficult it is to reverse the late consequences of unhealthy life-styles and behaviors. Once overt disease appears, it is usually necessary to supplement self-healing with the resources of the treatment model.

The effect of genetic predisposition and our environment on well-being is also indicated on the figure. A healthy genetic predisposition and healthy environment assist in the healing process. Although we cannot choose our genetic inheritance, we can have a powerful effect on whether these tendencies ultimately express themselves as disease. For example, whether a predisposition toward heart disease actually results in heart disease is strongly effected by how we care for our body (see chapter 6, the cardiovascular system). Unlike our genes, we can, within limits, choose our emotional and physical environment. Although limited in our ability to impact directly on the air we breathe (we can of course change where we live), we can take smaller steps such as creating more solitude in our lives and nurturing ourselves, as best as possible, with harmonious and balanced surroundings.

With practice and patience, mindfulness, can take us beyond the conventional definition of health, the absence of the sign or symptoms of disease, toward wholeness, the presence of wisdom, peace, harmony, and balance—perhaps we can call this "super health." The mind is still, the heart open, and we can see and experience what is happening in the here and now. Although we all touch into this feeling for brief moments, sustaining this feeling for a lifetime requires completion of all the steps in the healing program.

There will be many times when you attain moments of tranquility, well-being, and insight only to lose them in anger, distress, or irritation over an event of daily life. In such cases become mindful of what has happened and return to your practice. Mind-talk, its desires and the restless mind, do not give up easily. In the beginning, it will often seem like a battle between your good intentions and your old ways of thinking and behaving. When you get frustrated, discouraged, resistant, and are ready to give up, watch these feelings (they are also mind-talk), and return to your practice, resting in the knowledge that there is no path to a life of health and wholeness other than persistent focus and effort. In time, as you discover the peace and joy of health and wholeness, your faith and endurance will increase, and you will notice that you naturally orient yourself towards increasing amounts of formal (mindfulness training) and informal (mindfulness in daily life) practice.

You may wonder how this model for health and healing applies to the individual whose illness is predominantly physical, for example sickle cell anemia or cerebral palsy. Although there are those who would question whether any disease is predominantly physical, until we have evidence of the opposite, I find it important to proceed from the position that certain diseases are manifested predominantly in the body. To the extent that the mind is healthy, a self-healing program can be initiated. Healing, in these instances, is working with harmful attitudes in the same manner as previously described. It may or may not be possible to alter the symptoms and limitations of these diseases, but it is always possible to approach them from a perspective of emotional and spiritual health, which inevitably alters the impact of disease on one's well-being. Health and wholeness, as we have defined it, is a possibility for all individuals, healthy or ill. Some may be required to work hard to overcome physical limitations, while others may have to work hard to achieve healing within their mental limitations, which for many, can be no less disabling.

THE PROGRAM

Our initial attempts at self-healing are often sabotaged by our mind-talk. Full of enthusiasm, we try one thing and then another as our inner dialogue pushes us forward with its commentary: you are getting older; there is no time to waste; the better and quicker you practice, the sooner it will come; it is the right thing to do; it is now or never. Soon the commentary changes to: I cannot fit it in today; this is only making me more upset; there must be an easier way; I tried and failed again; I will try again next year when it will be a better time.

When we plant a seedling we do not tell it how quickly to grow or how it might look when it has matured. First, it is important to place it in the right soil, with the right sun exposure, in the right climate. If we plant it improperly, it cannot grow. We water it with the right amount of water, fertilize it, prune it at the right places, and stake it in the correct position, carefully and patiently being mindful of its needs. It is much the same with a self-healing program. We must first plant the seed, which is our intention to direct ourselves toward self-healing. This seed must be planted in the soil of consciously lived healthy habits and attitudes and nourished with appropriate daily practices. In their own time, our bodies will be healthier, our minds wiser, and our spirit stronger. Our task is to make the effort at practicing, taking small steps one at a time, and avoiding the self-defeating tendency for a fast quick push.

The following steps will assist you in initiating your own healing program. Although they are presented sequentially, you may find yourself moving back and forth with attention to those steps that are most important at a specific moment in your life. Familiarize yourself with these steps. Carry them in your mind as a new memory and, when possible, contemplate their deeper significance.

STEP 1: BELIEVING THAT THERE MUST BE A BETTER WAY

We begin new directions in life when we are convinced that the old directions no longer work. Some of us move quickly from one direction to another, a style that has both assets and limitations. Others suffer through repeated failures and frustrations before finally giving up and moving on. Whichever your style, you will not seriously undertake a new direction until you have abandoned faith in your previous path, the belief that it meets your long-term goals, and placed value on proceeding in a new way. As with any other life change, it will be done only when you are convinced it is possible and essential to your life. Until then you will play with these new practices rather than fully engage them.

Step 1 may be completed in a moment of personal insight that is often preceded by years of self-reflection punctuated by unsuccessful attempts at new directions. More likely, it will occur gradually following many years of accumulated frustration and denial as the treatment model, with its reliance on outside fixes, is slowly abandoned as the exclusive approach to health.

STEP 2: KNOWING THE DIFFERENCE BETWEEN TREATMENT AND HEALING

Treatment uses external agents (medications, surgery, and physical therapy) to manipulate the body for the purpose of reducing and eliminating the signs and symptoms of disease. Healing uses the natural capacities of the mind and body to resist disease and promote health and wholeness. Treatment focuses on disease, healing on health. Treatment is dominated by the professional, healing can be accomplished only by the individual. Each has its time and place.

If you wanted a delicatessen sandwich you would not go to a Chinese restaurant and, when refused, continue to demand that they provide you with what they clearly cannot produce. The same logic applies here. Have a realistic expectation of what each approach can accomplish, and use them to best meet your needs.

STEP 3: ESTABLISH AN ENVIRONMENT FOR HEALING

When seeking health, it is necessary to seek out healthy people and healthy environments. Early in the program, we may not have the power to remain focused on the new direction when confronted with the overwhelming negativity of unhealthy people or environments. At such times, when we cannot remain with the individuals or environment without losing our ability to practice our program, it is not appropriate to destroy our possibilities, but rather to let go and move on. There will be other times when our practice and the program is sufficiently well established that unhealthy people or environments will have less of an impact.

How do we identify healthy people and environments? We do so by looking within to feel how our mind and body react to different situations. We all know what good energy feels like. Calmness, quiet, and peace within your mind-body signify healing environments. Restlessness, "mind chatter," and disharmony indicate unbalanced environments.

STEP 4: UNDERSTANDING THE BASIC TECHNIQUES: MINDFULNESS AND SELF-REGULATION

As discussed throughout this book, mindfulness and self-regulation are the main components of a self-healing program. They are equivalent to the techniques of diagnosis and therapy in the conventional treatment model. The first two aspects of mindfulness, attention and concentration, enable us to develop the capacity to observe and learn carefully and precisely about our mind and body. With this skill, we can, at all times, be aware of the state of our mind and body applying, where indicated, appropriate and timely self-regulation. The third aspect, meditation, helps us to achieve wholeness.

The mindfulness technique is learned through the thirty-minute daily practice of mindfulness training (Exercise 3, chapter 3). Some individuals may learn this technique without further assistance. Others may require the help of a teacher. Those who have considerable difficulty in quieting the mind may initially need to use exercise or other relaxation techniques to quiet the body as a prelude to mindfulness training or attend a retreat that will provide an atmosphere of solitude and study.

Although you may experience some rewards immediately, do not get stuck in the newly discovered pleasure of tranquility. Remember that mindfulness training is not about pleasure, it is about understanding, knowledge, wisdom, and presence. Early in your training, you will begin to notice changes in your life: a quieter mind, clearer thinking, less reactivity to people and events, and deeper understanding of your mind and body. As you become more skilled, it is important not to limit mindfulness to the thirty-minute training session. The training is practice for daily living. Whether you are eating, driving, working on a special project, or talking to a friend, you can practice mindfulness, which is attention to the present moment.

Like mindfulness, self-regulation will, with practice, become a natural part of your daily life. Begin your practice of self-regulation by establishing attitudes and life-styles consistent with conscious living and choosing and learning one of the techniques for controlled breathing (Exercise #6, chapter 5). The value of controlled breathing is that you can use it at any time, without drawing attention to yourself, to quiet your mind and body and reestablish mindfulness. It is helpful to check your breathing intermittently during the day. Rapid, small-volume, coarse, chest breathing is characteristic of stress. If you notice this happening, begin controlled breathing. If you can stay with it for just a few minutes, stress will begin to reverse itself.

Because these techniques are central to a healing program, the importance of this step cannot be overemphasized. Further readings are recommended (see bibliography) and, as previously mentioned, guidance or support from others who have mastered this technique can be of considerable help (see resources).

STEP 5: BEGINNING CONSCIOUS LIVING

Even though our minds may resist, it is important to begin the program by consciously incorporating into our daily lives those attitudes and behaviors that will support our practice, create an atmosphere of good-will with other individuals, oppose unhealthy tendencies, and, through our persistent focus on these attitudes and behaviors, enhance our mindfulness training.

Chapter 7 lists some of the attitudes and habits that form an important part of conscious living. Start slowly by practicing and being attentive to one new practice a month. How does it affect your mind and body? What is your resistance to it? What is the nature of this resistance? How does it affect your relationships with others? How does it affect the restlessness of your mind? Does it, with time, become a more natural and preferred way of living? If it does it will soon become a new habit.

STEP 6: MASTERING MINDFULNESS

This step uses and fine-tunes the first two aspects of mindfulness: attention and concentration. These aspects of mindfulness enable us to observe our mind and body carefully and precisely, with detachment. Through self-observation we can discover the essential laws and truths of life and living. As an example, it is valuable to use this approach to understand our unhealthy psychologic mind-talk (also discussed in chapter 7). The process of shifting attitudes from unhealthy to healthy involves three steps: 1) identifying and observing unhealthy attitudes, in contrast to automatically reacting to them, 2) using attention and concentration to observe these attitudes, and 3) staying with the unpleasant feelings as you observe them, allowing time for insights to emerge. As you increase your understanding of these attitudes, they will have less and less power as you learn to watch them rather than react. In time, harmful attitudes will dissipate, leaving a space for the development of new and healthier ones.

Through the mindfulness training process, you have learned how to hold a focus by practicing with your breath. Using as an example the attitude of deprivation (see chapter 7), begin by directing and focusing your mind on this attitude when it arises. Avoid "running" from it by using one of the many avoidance techniques you may have mastered. Concentrate on it whenever you have time, and, if necessary, assign a specific time each day for more in-depth concentration. Concentration is different from obsession. It is not an attempt to analyze or judge these issues. Instead, the aim is to plant our questions and concerns in our "mindful mind" and patiently watch and observe them. Do not seek insight. Practice the process and insight will come by itself.

Although it may be difficult to learn how to watch an issue rather than become absorbed in analyzing it, the process of attention and concentration will allow you to penetrate deeper into your concerns and help you in developing a clear understanding of them. Initially you will observe their superficial aspects, and then you will proceed to their more subtle and intangible aspects and finally to their deeper sources. As we release ourselves from the pull of unhealthy mind-talk, our mind increasingly quiets, and we become more able to be mindful of each moment in our life responding appropriately and in a healthy manner to each person and situation. When this process is complete, depending on your skills and situation—it may take days, weeks, or longer, you will be released from the negativity and stress of harmful attitudes. For some individuals, it may be necessary to receive assistance from a guide who is skillful in using these techniques for this purpose. It requires time and patience to shift our attitudes, but with sustained effort it will happen.

STEP 7: MASTERING SELF-REGULATION

The first component of self-regulation, conscious living, has been discussed in Step 5. This step requires identifying which of the three applications—general relaxation, regulating the mind, and regulating the body—we need to address. Then we must learn and apply the appropriate practices. The capacity for self-regulation as we now know from studies in PNI, includes but is not limited to:

- controlling the workings of our mind through mindfulness
- conditioning our heart and lungs to work at increased efficiency
- directing our health through nutritional choices
- relaxing our bodies at will
- regulating our blood pressure, pulse, and respiration
- balancing our internal physiology and biochemistry
- enhancing the function of the immune system

Each of these daily self-regulatory practices has been discussed in previous chapters and illustrated through relevant exercises. Mastery of these skills, as with any other skill, requires time, sustained effort, and ardent interest.

STEP 8: MAINTAINING BALANCE

Faced with the challenges of daily life, and the natural changes that occur over the period of a lifetime, maintaining attention to our lives and control over our mind and body requires persistent practice of mindfulness and self-regulation and the choice of healthy friends, lovers, and environments. We all know how easy it is to be pulled from our center back into harmful attitudes and actions. Awareness of our mind-body will enable us to take the necessary steps that move us back to our healthy center.

For most individuals this means a retreat into quiet and silence during which it is possible to recenter and take inventory of the issues that have been the source of distress. For others, this may occur over a quiet weekend or during a regularly scheduled retreat. Each opportunity will further refine your skills, enhance your health, and offer you the possibility of releasing more "stuff."

It is easy to be mindful and focused in an isolated cabin at the beach or the mountains. The challenge is to do it in the midst of daily life. Ultimately, health should not be dependent on the environment or your associates. Mindfulness and self-regulation should allow you to maintain health in any situation. While we are all "learning" and "practicing" health, we need to provide ourselves with environments and human support that facilitate this process.

STEP 9: BREAKTHROUGH TO WHOLENESS

The first eight steps can move our lives from ill health to excellent health. It is appropriate for the few who venture this far to stop at this step. There are others, however, who have glimpsed at one moment or another, a further step, another way of living—wholeness. Wholeness, when fully achieved, does not require effort to sustain itself. It is a way of experiencing and being in life that is difficult to express in words. It may be easier for you to understand it by returning, if you can, to a time and place in your life (as we did in an earlier chapter) when everything was natural, flowing, abundant, and complete. You will likely ascribe this occurrence to the convergence of specific outer circumstances. You may be correct. The experience, however, is an inner experience that can be achieved and sustained for a lifetime independent of the outer situation.

The full and sustained experience of wholeness requires devotion and commitment to it as a life goal. There is no other way. The necessary requirements are a life of simplicity, good will, compassion, full health, and the ardent commitment to the third component of mindfulness, meditation. Meditation moves beyond a focus on an issue or object. It begins with a focus on that aspect of ourselves that has been doing all the observing we have been discussing in the preceding chapters. We can call that part of ourselves the observer. It goes further eventually to move beyond the *idea* of an observer to the direct experience of each moment, no pain, no pleasure, no life, no death, just the peace of life as it exists each moment.

Although only a few will reach this final state of consciousness, the remainder of us who follow this program, Steps 1–8, can lead lives of full health, living out our potential with happiness and joy, healthy relationships, and fruitful occupations. It is likely that we will increasingly experience moments of wholeness and, with effort, sustain these moments for longer and longer periods of our life. Perhaps with the wisdom of older age and a release from the urgency and passions of youth, wholeness may become a way of life.

STEP 9: SERVING OTHERS

As we heal and achieve higher levels of health, we begin to move from seeking to giving. In compassionate devotion to others, we serve and at the same time are served. In this process we experience ourselves at deeper levels, affirming life and giving life. We pass on the gift that we have earned through our efforts, and through the way we live our lives.

THE FIRST YEAR

- Firmly establish your daily thirty-minute mindfulness training practice. Even if you only start with ten-minute sessions, begin.
- Whenever and wherever possible, apply mindfulness to your daily activities.

- Three to six months into your practice, plan to attend a meditation retreat, preferably mindfulness meditation, that lasts a minimum of three days.
- Find, or start, a community of individuals that regularly practice meditation, preferably the mindfulness meditation you studied in this book, and practice with them at least once each month.
- For each of the next twelve months, choose one practice of conscious living (refer to chapter 7, pages 119 & 120), and carefully introduce and work with this practice in your daily life.
- At the beginning of the second month, choose one type of controlled breathing (Exercise 6, chapter 5), and incorporate it as the first ten minutes of your daily mindfulness training.
- At the same time, begin to check your breathing during the day, and, when necessary, practice several minutes of controlled breathing to reestablish balance in your mind and body.
- In the beginning of the third month, if there are no medical contraindications, begin a thirty-minute daily walking program (Alternatively, other exercise programs can be introduced, for example swimming, bicycling, or aerobic dancing.).
- On a monthly basis, reevaluate the status of your program.
- At the conclusion of twelve months, attend your second retreat and establish your next twelve-month program.

This program incorporates the main elements of a self-healing program. Carefully assess it (the activities and the time commitments), the strength of your intention, and the availability of any important resources. If you are not ready for all of it, then extend it out to two years and begin it more slowly. What is most important is to begin and to become mindful of your life now.

FIFTY WAYS TO BEGIN SELF-HEALING

1. Stop yourself for several moments each day and ask the question, "What is happening this moment, within me and outside of me?"
2. Identify a specific object or activity, for example, a clock, meal

time, the TV. Each time you see this object let it remind you to bring your attention to the present moment.

3. Scatter some colored dots around your house and work area. Every time you see one, bring your attention to the present moment. These dots or any other fixed object (desk, chair, refrigerator, TV) can serve to remind your to attend to the present moment.

4. Check your breathing several times a day, observing its charac-ter, and then take several complete breaths.

5. Each day, pick a simple activity (for example, tying your shoes, brushing your teeth, walking upstairs) and carefully observe and become mindful of this activity.

6. When you are ready, increase this to two, three, and more activities until you are mindful of as many of your daily activities as possible.

7. When your mind is active, stand back from it and, for a few moments, carefully observe it.

8. Commit one day to observing and discovering what activates your mind-talk.

9. When in a conversation with another individual, observe how carefully you listen or how distracted you may be, and then, if you have been distracted, return your attention to the present moment experience.

10. Pick a day and consciously observe your walking by walking slower and slower. Notice how you resist this and how your body slows down when you stick with it. If you cannot do it for an entire day, do it for ten-minute periods.

11. On another day pick a different activity and slow it down to observe it carefully.

12. Whenever you become anxious, overreactive, or too intense about a situation, stand back, observe it, take responsibility for it, and notice how you have colored the present with the past.

13. When you get angry, accept it as your anger and examine its sources.

14. Become aware that others are often different rather than wrong.

15. When you are ready to judge another person, stop, look at your discomfort with this person, and examine what it tells you about yourself.

16. When a situation becomes very intense, get some space and reflect quietly on it before reacting.

17. Eat at least one meal a day, or, if this is not possible then a portion of one meal, slowly and mindfully.

18. Eat what you need, not what you want.

19. When purchasing new items ask the questions. "Do I need this? Will this make my life simpler or more complex?" Keep a record of what you buy and review it at the end of the month. Do these items still seem necessary? Do they make your life simpler or more complex?

20. Stop for a few moments each day and observe how your body feels.

21. Check your muscle tension. Allow your shoulders to drop, your mouth to slightly open, and your facial muscles to relax.

22. Check your breathing. Is it erratic or smooth? Check how your stomach feels. Is your heart pounding or your mind running at full speed?

23. Check your "energy level." What is it on a scale of one to ten?

24. Begin a stretching and exercise program by stretching at brief intervals during the day and walking whenever possible.

25. Bring more quiet into your life. Take walks outside during lunch, shut off the TV, turn off the car radio, stay off the telephone, and have a quiet meal and evening.

26. When you get anxious, do not get busy. Instead, get quiet.

27. If possible, plan a weekend retreat, *alone.*

28. Spend one day a week, or, if not possible, a part of a day, quietly alone.

29. Take one day to practice silence, saying *only what is necessary.* Examine how much of your energy is exhausted with excess verbal activity.

30. Each week, take one of the examples of conscious living (balance, contentment, simplicity, honesty, harmlessness, solitude, and healthy life-styles) and observe the presence or absence of these qualities in your daily life.

31. Review your daily schedule and rearrange it to allow time for your healing activities.

32. Establish a daily journal to record your observations and progress with your healing program.

33. Examine whether your activities, friends, worksite, and living environment support your healing program.
34. Explore ways in which your worklife and worksite can be more satisfying and healing.
35. Develop a community of friends and co-workers who share your values and concerns about health.
36. Use this community and your relationships to examine yourself as you reflect your personality, attitudes, and actions off of others. View all your relationships as learning experiences.
37. Cultivate the capacity to set boundaries and say no to people and situations that do not facilitate your health.
38. Examine your behavior to see if it is motivated by the desire to avoid discomfort and anxiety. Avoidance rarely is a healthy way to work with unpleasant feelings.
39. Think about whether you give in order to receive or for the rewards that come from giving without any expectation of return.
40. When it comes to your health, observe whether your beliefs, thoughts, and actions are consistent. For instance, are your beliefs about simplifying your life consistent with your other thoughts and actions?
41. Remind yourself frequently of the feeling of full health—its joy and vitality.
42. Add playfulness to each day by allowing unstructured, "nonproductive" time to do things that please you and are fun.
43. Live fully each day and enjoy the healing process.

SEVEN SMALL STEPS

The remaining seven steps are for you to fill in. You can use the list above, or look towards your own daily experience to determine what would fit your needs and would be easily integrated into your daily life.

44.

45.

46.

47.

48.

49.

50.

CONCLUSION

These steps move us progressively from a focus on the external and physical aspects of disease, symptoms and detectable abnormalities of the mind-body systems, to the inner aspects of disease, the root causes that are discovered in our mind, unhealthy attitudes and stress, and finally to the discovery of a healthy spiritual life, which must be the foundation for emotional and physical well-being. This healing program is a program for body, mind, and spirit.

While working this program, remember that healing is not an all-or-nothing affair. At different times in our lives we enter and reenter the process of inner discovery and healing. There are bursts forward, plateaus, and, at times, setbacks. By holding the goal of physical, emotional, and spiritual well-being in your mind, you will slowly master the necessary skills and move with a steady pace towards healing.

Chapter 9

NAVIGATING
THE HEALTH-CARE
SYSTEM

THE PRECEDING CHAPTERS have presented the details of an innovative and comprehensive program for health and healing that can be used by all individuals irrespective of their current state of health. Those of us who explore this new approach to health, the integration of conventional medicine and the new approaches of mind-body healing, are pioneers in a new and largely uncharted terrain. Strengthened by our faith, values, and determination, we are moving forward without maps and frequently without societal support. This chapter will provide advice to help you to do the following: 1) avoid the pitfalls and road-blocks of a medical and social system that too frequently focuses on disease rather than health, 2) use the existing health-care system to support your healing program, 3) choose and create healing communities and healthy environments, and 4) realize that we can move beyond the current medical care system toward a new vision of health and healing.

171

THE HEALING RELATIONSHIP: PRACTITIONER AND CLIENT

There are many who call themselves healers but very few whose sensitivities, knowledge, and training are adequate for the task. We are too frequently required to choose between well-educated medical scientists, whose training in the technological aspects of disease does not include an understanding of the healing process and the deeper sources of health and disease, and a multitude of "alternative healers" whose skills and capacities are difficult to evaluate. The following guidelines will help you to identify a health professional that can assist you, when necessary, in your healing program. It is important to remember that we are just now beginning to lay the groundwork for the training of a new kind of health professional. Living as we do in the midst of major change, it may be necessary for you to improvise, which may at times require you to "train" your health professional. Here, then, are the questions to ask when you look for a health professional:

DOES THE HEALTH PROFESSIONAL *WORK* AND *LIVE* ACCORDING TO A BASIC PHILOSOPHY THAT INCLUDES THE FOLLOWING BELIEFS?

- The goal of healing is full health. Full health is the individual's capacity to access and engage the many possibilities of his or her existence living and serving with peace, joy, love, and freedom.
- Every individual is a physical, spiritual, and emotional being. Healing must include all of these aspects of our lives.
- Through the use of mindfulness and self-regulation, every individual has the capacity for self-healing. Ultimately, it is the *individual* who is responsible for his own healing. The professional, through his or her words and actions must support the self-healing process.
- The individual must be involved directly in all aspects of the healing process. The role of the healer is to serve as a resource and guide.
- Each individual has unique talents, capacities, and life rhythms. The healer respects and works within the unique context of the individual's life.

IS THE HEALER WELL-TRAINED IN THE TECHNIQUES OF HEALING?

A healing perspective, as outlined above, does not substitute for skill. Although this book outlines an approach to healing that uses the techniques of mindfulness and self-regulation, many other techniques may be of value for particular individuals in particular circumstances. What is important is that the healer's skills assist the individual in achieving the capacity for self-healing. However appropriate the skills of the healer, if these are not practiced in a manner that supports self-healing, the result will ultimately be "treatment," not "healing."

IS THE HEALER DEEPLY COMMITTED TO HIS OR HER OWN HEALING?

It is not possible for you to be guided toward a higher level of healing than is already present in the life of the healer that serves as your guide.

IS THE HEALER COMPASSIONATE, OPEN, COMMUNICATIVE, PATIENT, KIND, AND AVAILABLE?

I have provided these ideas realizing that individuals cannot control the actions of health professionals, but they can, however, seek to choose professionals whose emphasis is on listening, caring, and nonintervention (i.e., not relying on drugs, diagnostic testing, and surgery). Being mindful of what you are looking for will best guarantee your success. Your physician is not a mind-reader (although he/she, as with many of us, often thinks he/she knows what others want). Your physician will treat you as he or she is trained and accustomed to. If you want something different, ask!

Using the above guidelines, meet with your prospective health provider before you make a final decision. As you would with a conventional physician, ask how certain problems would be handled, how long office visits are, how accessible he or she is, observe the office setting, the staff, and do not forget to check on training. If he or she is uncomfortable with your questions, you need to try someone else. As with most relationships, it may take time and effort to find the one that suits you. When you do, use that person as a resource for your program, and do not be pulled into the practitioner's idea of how you should run your life.

Is it possible to integrate and sustain a healing perspective along these lines in a conventional healing practice—particularly in a practice defined as a medical practice? This is the question I asked myself as I left a large HMO to explore if and how it would be possible to practice humanistic medicine and holistic healing within the constraints of the well-established health-care system.

The answer is yes. With creativity and patience, it is not only possible, but also practical and desirable to practice this new approach to health and healing. Several key elements make it possible.

- The character of the practice must express and be guided by the values outlined above.
- All staff members must share these values and perspectives.
- There must be the luxury of time to listen to each individual, perform the needed diagnostic evaluations, and teach and practice with the client the techniques of mindfulness and self regulation. In my practice, I schedule no appointment for less than thirty minutes. Even when the actual time needed is less, I adhere to this policy. I maximize my interaction with individuals by returning all telephone calls, directly performing any necessary testing, and by minimizing the use of other helpers. Each of these segments of time allows more time to talk, listen, and know each other.
- As health insurance carriers do not reimburse for time spent talking, so called "cognitive-time," both health professionals and clients must be flexible and innovative when it comes to payment. Although far from resolving this dilemma, I have partially succeeded by 1) assisting my clients in obtaining health insurance that compensates for "prevention", 2) exploring and understanding the definitions and limits of billing insurance companies, 3) accepting less monetary reimbursement for my time, and 4) minimizing my expenses (I have no receptionist, no billing clerk, use a secretary four to eight hours each week, and sublet space in my office to other physicians), and 5) expecting my clients to be willing to expend additional financial resources on prevention and education.

A number of organizations can assist you in finding a "holistic provider," but, in searching it is important to consider the above guidelines. Unfortunately, because the term holistic has come to mean many things to many people, nothing can replace your personal judgment and experience.

HEALTH INSURANCE—
OR SHOULD WE CALL IT "DISEASE INSURANCE"?

This section is directed toward those who have the option of choosing among various health insurance policies or programs. (The thirty million Americans who do not have this option, although they are capable of self-care, are a shameful reminder of the deficiencies of our system.)

The term "health insurance" is a misnomer. Rarely do health insurers cover the cost of healing and prevention services. When they do, as in the case of some HMO and conventional insurers, the coverage is minimal. The reasons, which are incredibly shortsighted are that 1) most individuals, as a result of job turnover, carry a specific policy for the short term, one to five years; however, the results of a prevention and healing program accumulate over many years and are not reflected in the immediate corporate "bottom line," and 2) the outcome of prevention and healing programs, which are not exclusively limited to improving physical well-being but include the discovery of peace, joy, and personal growth, are neither measurable through a microscope nor considered directly relevant to health. We are left with expensive policies that only reimburse for conventional medical diagnostic and treatment programs.

Confronted with this reality, I have incorporated several possible solutions into my life and professional practice. These include the following: 1) selecting health insurance that offers the best opportunity for prevention and healing services, 2) using and interpreting existing health insurance policies to their limits, 3) using the free or reduced-cost services of organizations that teach techniques of self-healing, 4) becoming more self-reliant, 5) learning from friends, and 6) allocating more of my personal resources towards self-healing.

The rapidly changing health insurance field is so complex that I find it necessary and helpful to explain the options to my clients. To begin, your options are often limited by the choices presented to you by your employer. If you want options with more preventive and healing coverage, investigate the full range of available health insurance coverage, and "lobby" for the best one with your benefits office. When preventive services are not available through any of the insurance options, you can lobby for the company itself to offer some of these services directly (see section on worksite) on-site, a policy gaining increasing acceptability in the corporate world.

There are two major options: 1) traditional health insurance, through which you select the health provider of your choice whose covered services are reimbursed by the insurance company and 2) the HMO, which is of two sorts—the "fixed panel" and the "open panel"—the former, of which Kaiser Permanente is an example, employs or contracts with a group of physicians you are obligated to use, usually at a central location. In the latter, the "open panel" the HMO offers you a choice of a variety of community physicians who practice in their existing offices.

Each of these approaches has its advantages and disadvantages. Neither go very far in covering healing-related services. This problem is built into the system in two ways. Firstly, the system, as previously discussed, is oriented toward disease care. Secondly, and most importantly, the reimbursement system primarily compensates "procedures" at the expense of "talking time." As an example, an insurance company will pay, without question, $450 for a twenty-minute procedure that consists of passing a tube through the mouth and into the stomach for a view of a potential ulcer, while at the same time often denying, or minimally compensating for, the time necessary to talk about the sources of the ulcer and to work with mindfulness and self-regulatory techniques to eradicate this problem for the long term.

Having worked with each of these plans, I can offer one final thought. Although the HMO offers the advantage of pre-paid care with no insurance forms, and the fixed panel often provides in-house educational programs, it is important to know that the providers have no control over their schedules and the amount of time they spend with each individual. In reality, they are expected to follow guidelines that require that they see twelve to fifteen patients in a 3.5-hour span of time. This allows, with paper work and telephone calls, less than ten minutes on the average per person. The private practice physicians, as they increasingly sign up for the open panel HMO and preferred provider organization (PPO) are forced to see more patients to compensate for the reduced payment through these systems. The result is a problem in either case, but the private physician still maintains a flexibility not available to the the fixed panel HMO physician. In either case, the situation does not encourage healing.

When choosing a plan consider the following issues:

- Does it compensate for routine preventive health examinations? This time allows at least one yearly compensated session that can be used for prevention and healing-related activities.
- What is its mental health coverage? As strange as it seems, mental health coverage also offers an opportunity for the creative practitioner to use reimbursed time for healing activities.
- Does it reimburse for alternative approaches? These may include biofeedback, body work, acupuncture, music and drama therapy.
- Does it allow you sufficient flexibility to choose a health-care professional that shares your values?
- Does your plan provide or reimburse for health-related educational activities?
- Does your plan offer financial incentive for healthy life-styles?

GETTING THE MOST FROM YOUR INSURANCE

I have discovered that, whatever the insurance plan, if I am willing to be creative, I can usually "expand" the covered services to include at least part of the time necessary for healing work. I am sharing these ideas with you to assist you and your provider to maximize the benefits available to you.

Using the approach of self-healing, it is still possible to be reimbursed ethically. For me, the appropriate self-healing program for most illness includes acquiring an understanding of the sources of the illness through mindfulness techniques and the capacity to use self-regulation for healing and health promotion. This approach requires several office visits to introduce, teach, and practice these healing techniques with the client. Each of these visits is a legitimate form of "medical treatment" for the specific problem brought to my attention by the client. The difference is that I have chosen to heal it, at its source, through techniques that work at that level. Because the reimbursement system pays for the office management of a medical condition, it is possible to be reimbursed for mindfulness and self-regulatory training. This is both ethical and appropriate, heals the client, and ultimately offers significant cost savings for the insurance carrier.

I extend this approach to include a variety of self-regulatory techniques including biofeedback, relaxation training, imagery, and nutrition services. For example, hypertension is partly the result of an overactive sympathetic circulation, which is responsive to biofeedback and other forms of self-regulatory training. My view of health permits me to consider these services to be part of the "treatment" of hypertension. That is how I categorize them for insurance purposes.

When mental health benefits are available, I use them within the healing perspective; that is, all disease (hypertension, migraines, coronary heart disease, ulcer disease, colitis, etc.) are either initiated or exacerbated by unhealthy mental attitudes, which are most effectively and efficiently healed through the techniques of mindfulness and self-regulation.

All of these are inadequate and unfortunate ways to use a disease-oriented insurance system that has become bankrupt through its own policies of excessively compensating procedures and treatment at the expense of healing. It is sad that we must work so hard for reimbursement for healing services from a system that sells itself as "health insurance." When we have exhausted its possibilities, we must turn to other sources.

THE WORKSITE

Corporations are finally becoming aware of the high cost of their policies and practices. It has been estimated that sixty to ninety percent of all physician office visits are for stress-related disorders.[1] The California Workman's Compensation Institute reports that stress-related claims have increased 434 percent between 1982 and 1986.[2] The

National Council on Compensation Insurance estimates that compensation claims related to stress account for fourteen percent of all claims, a figure that is considerably underestimated and certain to rise.[3] Corporations pay the price tag through their expenditures on employee health insurance, which accounts for twenty-five percent of the total health care expenditures, almost $150 billion per year.

The causes of worksite stress are apparent to all: long hours, excessive out-of-town travel, endless "crisis management," dead-end jobs, job instability, inadequate or nonexistent supervisor-employee communication, lack of involvement in decision-making, unhealthy facilities, and the modern-day phenomenon of mergers and takeovers, which leave the average worker with uncertainty and, at worst, without a job.

The preceding chapters have clearly stated the viewpoint that we are each responsible for what happens to our mind and body. In our routine day-to-day life, it is often difficult, however, to resist the effects of a stressful and unhealthy work environment. Individuals feel trapped with few choices except to surrender helplessly to worksite stress or leave their jobs, which may be a financial impossibility.

Corporations live with the results of their styles. These include high absenteeism, low productivity, high turnover, job accidents, and increased health and disability claims. When the bottom line is affected, management starts paying attention. The result is a new and growing concern for worksite stress reduction and health promotion. A 1985 survey of corporations with more than fifty employees indicated that from fifteen to sixty percent of these had some form of stress-management programs. When the survey broadened the perspective to include any form of health promotion activity, two-thirds of the corporations indicated a direct involvement in health promotion.[4]

This offers each of us new options in navigating ourselves into relatively stress-free work environments. It is important, however, to be aware of the paradox that management often fails to take the essential step of looking at its own practices, so even if they provide stress management courses, employees may face the added stress of more clearly seeing that some of the problem is within the corporate style, and this aspect may be less amenable to change.

Individuals with a personal commitment to health and healing must consider whether their employer's attitude and actions reflect a concern for the health and well-being of their employees and consider this an important criteria in selecting a worksite. The following are useful questions to ask before accepting a new position:

- Is there a human services office?
- Is there an Employee Assistance program (EAP)? These programs are of two types. Some are limited to problems related to alcohol and substance abuse. Others, called broad brush, are expanded to include other mental health concerns. What are the administrative policies for employees found to be suffering from alcohol and substance abuse? This will tell you a great deal about a company's attitude toward employees.
- Are there health promotion programs? Of what type? Would your family be included? Who pays the cost? Would you do the program on your time or their time?
- Will they reimburse you for outside health promotion programs?
- Is there a fitness facility or showers?
- Is there a "quiet room"?
- Do the health insurance options cover prevention and mental health?
- Are there windows, adequate ventilation, greenery, and quiet workspaces?
- What is the attitude and policy regarding overtime?
- What are the vacation benefits?

The more we value our health, the more we will consider these issues as central to our job choices. The concern for health promotion is rapidly moving through the corporate world so you and your co-workers and union can use your influence to coax your personnel or human services department into allocating resources (time or money) toward these programs.

Unfortunately many of us do not as yet have the options of an enlightened corporation. Even after we have made the best available choice, burnout from stress can occur. Our option at this point is to re-examine what can be done to improve the worksite environment, consider the possibility of other employment, and simultaneously use this opportunity to work with mindfulness and self-regulation. When stress has progressed to the level that it disables the individual from effective performing of work, the approach is direct and simple.

- I provide an opportunity for an individual to take a break of one to four weeks from the worksite. In order to assure no loss of income, when possible, I provide the individual with a certificate for sick leave or disability. It is not necessary to wait for physical illness to emerge, and it is infrequent that the corporation questions the cause for "leave." I have discovered considerable opportunity, particularly in large corporations, to use employee's benefits in this manner. I believe "mental health days" are essential in certain circumstances—if they must be called "sick days" or "disability," I comply with this need. This again is an unfortunate, but necessary, way to work with the legitimate needs of people.
- During this leave I assist the individual in structuring a period of rest and recuperation. Removal from the stressful setting often results in a quieter mind and the capacity to see things in a new and fresh way. Decisions can be made and options can be reevaluated as the heart and soul regain their spirit.
- When the immediate crisis has subsided, I introduce mindfulness and self-regulation techniques. The use of relaxation techniques, biofeedback, exercise, yoga, and proper nutrition can assist with increasing resistance to stress and introducing more balance into life.
- Finally, we begin to reevaluate plans and goals for the future.

For individuals suffering lesser levels of stress, a modification of this program is appropriate. The central point is that it is possible for an individual, either directly or with the assistance of a supportive health provider, to 1) choose to work for corporations that are actively concerned with worksite stress and health promotion, 2) influence a corporation to begin worksite health promotion programs, and 3) successfully use existing worksite benefits to advantage in pursuing a healing program. None of us are helpless in navigating the issue of worksite stress. Until our society accepts health and healing as a major life value, our quest for health will frequently be in opposition to the practices and policies of the corporate world.

HEALING COMMUNITIES

One of the most difficult challenges of healing is to maintain tenacity of purpose in the face of popular wisdom, entrenched corporate management styles, and a system of health care that appears incapable of adjusting to prevention and health-promotion approaches. Individuals who share these views and directions are a source of knowledge, inspiration, support, and nurturing.

As a society, we place such high value on individuality and independence that we have largely lost the personal capacity to join and share with other individuals. The result is the loss of the nurturing, support, and continuous nonjudgmental feedback necessary for self-growth that is characteristic of healthy communities of two or more people. From our earliest moments in life we learn from and experience our lives through others. We are social animals, and it can be no other way. We cannot change ourselves or the world by ourselves. Other individuals are essential for health and healing. We can open ourselves to the healing power of community and relationship by examining our attitudes and approaches to close relationships (see section on loneliness, chapter 7), by developing the skills necessary for healing relationships, and by seeking out like-minded groups of individuals.

Building healing relationships is an art and skill. Many of these issues are discussed in chapter 7. Honest intimate relationships force us to see ourselves, confront our unhealthy attitudes and actions, and rediscover the openness and love that is at the core of our being. Communities can range from the two-person intimate relationship, to groups of friends, support groups, self-help groups, task-oriented groups, and groups that come together over shared interests and ideals.

For a group to transform and sustain itself as a *healing* community, it must adhere to certain specific practices and values. These include a commitment to

- free and open sharing of feelings
- honesty, authenticity, confidentiality, and trust
- patience, listening, and nonjudgment of others
- equality among group members

- the resolution of conflict through dialogue and negotiation
- health and healing

The power and success of a healing community such as Alcoholics Anonymous is based on the effective and unalterable use of the above principles. The same can be said of healthy friendships, intimate relationships, or any other community that lives through these principles. If you maintain these ideas through your personal actions, it is inevitable that your communities will become healing communities, and you will have created a valuable tool in navigating yourself toward full health.

HEALING ENVIRONMENTS

As we structure our environments, our environments in turn structure our lives. Similar to a healing community, a healing environment is essential for health and well-being. A healthy individual and a healthy environment are inseparable. Without clean water and air, an appropriate use of our natural resources, and maintenance of our soil and forests, health and human life are impossible.

The concern for our environment must also extend to our created environments. As a culture, we are often insensitive to the importance of our surroundings. As an example, consider the hospital setting, which is supposed to be an intensive healing environment. The rooms are impersonal, sterile, and cold, the windows rarely offer an uplifting view, the atmosphere is serious and intense, the wards are noisy, the rooms are illuminated with harsh fluorescent lighting, the staff is busy and harried, the food lacks "life and love," the gowns are standardized and required, and the patient has little control over his or her time or the decisions regarding his or her life as he or she is poked and probed with few explanations and less sensitivity. Everyone tries, but the result is an environment conducive to treatment not healing.

Unfortunately the same is too often true of our daily living environments. Although none of us are completely free to create our living space, we have considerably greater opportunity than we are willing to acknowledge or act upon. This opportunity can be maximized if we approach our day-to-day life with mindfulness and the intent to create a healing environment through self-regulatory actions. Ask the following questions:

- Is my life cluttered with activities and possessions that I do not need?
- Do I feel quiet, calm, and peaceful in my home? If not, how can I create a healing atmosphere?
- Do the stores at which I shop at (e.g. shopping malls versus smaller stores) and the streets I drive on support healing?
- Does the music I listen to, do the clothes I wear, does the food I eat support healing?
- Do my daily pace and rhythm support healing?
- Do the pace and rhythm of my speech, eating habits, sleep, and exercise style support healing?
- Have I maximized the ability to create a healing atmosphere in my home and at the worksite?
- Do I have a special "sacred" space to which I can go when I need solitude?
- Do my friends, lovers, coworkers, and other acquaintances support my healing intention?
- Does my inner environment support healing?

It would be valuable to use the mindfulness technique to focus your attention for one week on each of these issues, exploring their deeper significance in your daily life. Holding these ideas in your mind, you can slowly create an image of your ideal environment and begin to make it happen in your daily life.

There is much we can all do to go around or through the environmental hazards in our life to create a healing space, but we will soon notice the limitations of our personal actions when confronting a global environment that is "sick" and in much need of healing. We cannot and should not avoid the reality that the industrial and technologic revolutions have, in a brief few centuries (the first producing oil well was drilled only one hundred years ago), caused irreparable damage to the earth and its life forms. If this destruction does not cease, there will be little sense in discussing the possibilities of personal healing. It will not be possible. Ultimately healing is a process we must all do together, at all levels, personal and global.

THE HEALING SELF

We must, of course, ultimately return to ourselves, the navigators and authors of our own lives. Although we are forever searching outside for answers, we remain our own first and best available resource. Through the use of mindfulness we can uncover this resource, and, through self-regulation, use it. Read the following questions, but do not try to answer them immediately.

- Do you believe in your self-healing capacities? Do your actions reflect your words and thoughts?
- Do you spend more time *talking about* your health or *doing something about it*?
- Are you trained in, or planning to be trained in, mindfulness and self-regulatory techniques?
- Do you prefer to be healthy or financially secure? These are not necessarily exclusive of each other, but sometimes you may have to make a choice.
- Do you choose health over unhealthy relationships and unhealthy jobs?
- Does your daily living environment reflect your health values?
- Are you too busy to become healthy?
- Do you need to be sick before you can become well?

Although we all know the "right" answers to these questions, our actions all too often do not reflect this knowledge. If we are ever to experience full health, we must become aware of our intended actions *before* we act. The brief moment of time between the intention to act and the action must be extended to allow sufficient time for mindfulness. Only in this way can we be free to choose our actions rather than automatically reacting according to our inner program. So rather than answer the above questions in words, it is more appropriate to answer them with actions.

Each time we act in a manner that is consistent with our beliefs we feel a sense of inner cohesiveness. When our actions are inconsistent with our beliefs we experience inner conflict. It is at such moments that we recognize that the path to healing is not an easy one. We need whatever help we can get, and we must recognize that we do not live and cannot be healed isolated from the larger community. Our ability to attain and sustain full health invariably is influenced by the character of our health-care system, the values and practices of our culture, families, and employers, and the health of our planet. New approaches to health and healing require that we reexamine our values and institutions.

BEYOND ACCOMMODATION

We take a much longer and less certain road to health and healing when we consume our energies accommodating to an outmoded and limited health-care system and societal values and practices that are more conducive to disease than health. Rather than moving forward, we too often feel as if we are constantly defending ourself against the careless destruction of our living environment, the harmful effects of jobs that offer little meaning and much stress, the numbing effect of an educational system that teaches facts without values, the despair of failed relationships, and the powerlessness that, for very real reasons, permeates the lives of so many. We need a new vision.

Those who think on a global and national level, envisioning the political, economic, and social world of the future, and those who think on a more individual level, envisioning the possibilities for human growth and development, would agree that personal health and healing is the basis for sustained change in our global, national, and personal lives. It is within this context that the preceding chapters have presented the fundamental principles of health and healing: mindfulness and self-regulation. It is through the mastery of these approaches to living that we can arrive at an understanding of the nature of our lives and existence and act with sensitivity, wisdom, and freedom in the world about and within us. In this way we can live with the peace and love necessary to create a local, national, and global reality that reflects our inner truth.

Living as we do in an "in-between" time, it is often necessary to work within the existing framework as we leap forward and create new approaches that more clearly meet our needs. The accommodations and energy that are necessary to do this can deaden the soul and divert us from the important task ahead. This chapter outlines the reality of navigating through a system that no longer works.

Having attempted to stretch the existing system as far as possible to accommodate a broader vision of health and healing, I am convinced that it is necessary to step out of this system and create a new model that takes the best of contemporary medicine and enhances and expands it with the practices, techniques, and human experiences that characterize a broader vision of health, healing, and the possibilities of human life. The time has come to move our visions out of our minds and into reality.

Serving as an oasis for those whose energies are depleted by the stress of living in an unhealthy society, and as an experiment that incorporates the principles of mind-body healing and ecological living, the emerging health center of tomorrow reaches backward to incorporate many of the principles of Aesclepian and yogic healing and forward to implement the new and exciting research of psychoneuroimmunology. It is about to become a reality. What will this new health center look like?

THE CENTER FOR MIND-BODY HEALING

Much like the Aesclepian healing temples of ancient Greece, the healing center of tomorrow will be removed from the frenetic pace of day-to-day city life. It will be set in nature, a reminder and a mirror through which we can rediscover the natural pace, rhythms, and seasons of life. Scaled to a "human size" the center will be a home away from home, a place to live, eat, work, play, reflect, learn, and *heal*—a time to recapture one's energies, share in community, re-envision the future, experience the feeling of aliveness, and master the capacity for mindfulness and self-regulation.

The staff will model, practice, and teach the principles of health and healing. Music, drama, the visual arts, exercise, body work, healthy nutrition, service work, play, meditation, imagery, yoga and other healing modalities will be used to assist the healing process. Of course, when appropriate, the brilliant technologies of contemporary medicine, within the healthful context of the healing center, will also be utilized.

Some will come to the center for rest and renewal, others will come seeking relief from specific medical disorders. Some may stay for a few weeks, and others will stay for longer periods, seeking the opportunity for a deeper and more complete healing. The center will respond to each individual's unique needs. It will be neither a treatment center nor a "holistic," or "spiritual" center. It will be a healing center, which will incorporate all the aspects of the human experience, mind, body, and spirit.

The natural questions will arise—"Is it possible?" "How will this be paid for?" Models already exist that have demonstrated the practicality of this approach, and the willingness of individuals to expend the necessary personal and economic resources to bring peace, joy, and fulfillment into their lives. The cost of health and healing is ultimately far less than the cost of treating disease, recovering from broken relationships, and living in despair. What are the alternatives?

The model I am proposing will offer each of us the opportunity for a richer, more peaceful, and joyous life. It will offer health professionals a release from the pressures of a failed system. It will offer corporations healthier and more productive employees, and it will offer our society an affordable alternative to the existing bankrupt system. There is much work ahead.

In this chapter I have attempted to create a bridge between the world of health care in which we now live and through which we must navigate, and the promise and vision of a different set of values and institutions that we are about to create with each of our lives. We must be patient and persistent in this quest for health. Each step into the future is challenging, a bit uncertain, and, at times, fearful. When the task ahead seems too large, I remember a short story told by Joseph Campbell. "During the 1960s," he related, "after I had addressed a large audience, a young woman, no more than twenty years, old came up to me and said, 'Mr. Campbell, my generation no longer needs to spend the years journeying towards the wisdom and understanding of life that you have achieved. We can "get it" at a young age.' "I looked at her," he stated, "and said, 'That's wonderful—all you have missed is life.'" It is a lesson we must all learn as we navigate our lives and our culture towards healing and health.

Chapter 10

THE FOUR STAGES
OF HEALING

There is something irreversible about the healing process. Once begun, like a fruit that has ripened and can no longer return to its unripened condition, we can not reverse its course. Knowledge, growth, and healing have a compelling quality that, once experienced, becomes undeniable. Those who choose to awaken, and through sustained and sometimes painful efforts at healing engage the many possibilities and capacities of their existence, will invariably be released from the fetters of their programming and dis-ease and be free to live self-directed lives. Those past and present explorers who have engaged this process have described in many different languages and forms the personal, and at the same time universal, journey to health and healing. As with all essential truths the basic elements of this journey remain unchanged through the ages.

THE FIRST STAGE OF HEALING:
WORKING WITH SYMPTOMS

Whether it be Adam thrust from the Garden, Oedipus driven from Thebes, Parsifal ejected from the castle, or you and I experiencing sudden crisis in our well-ordered lives, the first stage of healing always begins with breakdown. It may be as subtle as the slow, almost imperceptible appearance of physical or emotional distress or as dramatic as the sudden pain of a heart attack. It may be initiated by the loss of a loved one, the end of an important relationship, occupational burnout, or the malaise and boredom that too often comes with financial and occupational "success."

Suddenly, we are awakened from a deep sleep and drawn into a relationship with our distress. Our control gives way to fear, the gridlock of time bursts open and time, never available for health maintenance, is now readily available for disease care. Daily demands are suspended, and our focus shifts from the known to the unknown. We become intensely sensitive to our longing for, and the fragility of, life and the importance of loved ones.

This first stage of healing is characterized by a focus on, and attention to, the external manifestations of distress; symptoms and detectable abnormalities of the mind-body's systems (as discussed in chapter 8, Steps 1–4). Physicians are sanctioned by society as the appropriate guides through the important process of diagnosis and treatment. We all know the ritual, and I want to emphasize its importance. The traditional medical history, physical and diagnostic examination, and treatment program are essential components of a comprehensive healing program.

We must not misconstrue the role of conventional medicine in a comprehensive healing program to mean that scientific medicine is flawed and inadequate. None of us would return to a time when medicine lacked the brilliance and high technology that it has today. No one who has looked at a CAT scan or MRI, watched the life-saving practices of trauma medicine, had a relative who received an organ transplant, or recovered through skillful surgery or the appropriate use of antibiotics will deny the wonder of modern medicine. It is not flawed; it is limited.

Some, however, will hear no further call and remain satisfied with the familiarity and achievements of the conventional approaches to health. They choose to stay within the known, accepted, and tested methods of the "higher authority" of medicine. These individuals are either un-aware of or uninterested in the possibility of a more comprehensive and permanent healing. They may offer many excuses for their unwilling-ness to pursue a deeper healing: "I do not have enough time." "I do not have enough money." "I am too busy this week." "I am feeling better." "My insurance will not cover it. Are you sure it works?"

Others hear a voice from within saying, "There must be more—there must be a better way." It is these individuals who will discover and use the techniques of mindfulness and self-regulation and shift from a *dependence* on health professionals to a *collaboration* with them and finally to an emphasis on self-reliance and self-directed change. They frequently experience an immediate and sustained improvement and, in some cases, with patience and persistence, the elimination of the troubling disorder. Their balance is restored, they learn important new lessons in self-reliance, develop essential lifetime skills, and create the possibility that health and healing can become a constant and central focus of their lives. The discussions in the earlier chapters of this book can help you achieve this important first phase of healing.

THE SECOND STAGE OF HEALING: HEALING AT THE SOURCE

The second phase of healing (see chapter 8 Steps 5–7) requires that we further extend our use of mindfulness and self-regulation to assist in shifting our focus from the *outer* aspects of distress to an exploration of its *inner* sources. Expanding on the first phase of healing, we penetrate deeper into the distress seeking a knowledge of its essential meaning from which deeper lessons are learned, wisdom gained, and healing completed.

This stage of healing requires silence. As the ancients have taught us, deeper understanding of the human experience can only be achieved individually, in solitude. It requires dedicated time each day to observe and explore, through mindfulness, the inner aspects of our lives. The use of concentration, the second component of mindfulness, is a particularly valuable resource for this stage of healing (as discussed in chapter 7). If possible, a silent retreat would be of value at the onset of this process and at selected times during it. Although this essential work must be done in solitude, it can be of considerable help to seek the assistance of a guide who is familiar with the various stages of healing. You will likely discover that, when you are ready, the teacher has a strange way of appearing.

This second phase of healing is often called a "separation." Our shift from a preoccupation with the outer aspects of distress to a focus on the inner, underlying aspects of the disorder manifests itself as a partial withdrawal from the outer world. As we transfer our energy to inner demands we may have to say no to outside demands. Each progressive insight offers new challenges, sources of energy, and life direction. Life, previously a struggle, moves towards a natural flow. Relationships troubled by conflict become more harmonious. Distress is increasingly perceived as a condition that results from the effects of ignorance, blindness, and limited consciousness of the mind and body.

The uncovering of these more obscure layers of experience is how we continue on the healing path. At this point, we begin to see how important it is to be committed to what we are doing and how much discipline and faith are necessary in the process of healing. Although we are only at the second phase of healing, few individuals come this far, and we should feel some sense of achievement for arriving at this difficult stage. This phase of healing may take one month, one year, or ten years. For some, it is only a brief encounter with the possibility of a deeper healing, which will be renewed should distress reemerge. For others, it is incorporated as an ongoing focus of life, a continuing exploration of the unknown territory of the self.

THE THIRD STAGE OF HEALING:
WISDOM, WHOLENESS, AND FULL HEALTH

It is the unusual individual who passes through and completes the second stage of healing. It is even rarer for an individual to go further. The third stage of healing (see chapter 8, Step 8) is not about healing distress and disease (which occurs in the second stage of healing), it is about uncovering a fundamental, comprehensive, and unchanging knowledge that displaces all previous ways of knowing and understanding life—a knowledge of the depths that conveys a more profound understanding of the surface. The veils begin to lift, and we move away from the preoccupation with the appearances and forms of the outside world and our inner perceptions with their separateness and distinctiveness, and we move toward an inner experience of an elemental formlessness, connectedness, wholeness, and union with all aspects of life.

With an outer life that emphasizes purity of heart, clarity of perception, proper attitudes, appropriate action, inexhaustible courage, a resolute aspiration for healing, and the steady, persistent practice and application of mindfulness training, our consciousness expands. As we describe this stage of healing we begin to become lost in our words. Healing, at this level, becomes known and understood only in proportion to which it is directly experienced by the individual. Language has been developed to describe, explain, and communicate the more objective and external aspects of life. There are, however, aspects that cannot be communicated through words. The deeper experience of self, wholeness, completeness, and the more profound and subtle understanding of life is one of those elusive aspects. It is appropriate to honor this reality and stop here, leaving a further comprehension of this phase of healing to those who venture this far and directly experience its nature.

Although we lack the words to describe adequately this experience, at this level of healing, we achieve the most profound fruits of a program of mindfulness and self-regulation: mental and physiologic peace. Stress, and its fears and anxieties, no longer need to be managed or controlled—they are gone. Gone with it are all of its chemical messages to the body that distort and imbalance our physiology. Powerlessness, loneliness, and deprivation, distressful attitudes and the associated misperceptions of a mind that dwells through its endless profane mind-talk on what never was, will not require further analysis, self-affirmations, workshops, or drugs.

What remains will be a mind-body that functions as it was born to function—in perfect balance and harmony, joy, and delight through the years that are given to each of us. No doubt, as a normal result of the aging of our mind-body and the untoward effects of an unhealthy environment, we will all, at one time or another, supplement mindful-ness and self-regulation with the marvels of modern scientific technol-ogy. This is considerably different from the persistent, increasing, and inappropriate dependency on health professionals and their technology that can bankrupt a system that neither uses nor understands the essential resources required for a deeper healing: self-reliance, mindful-ness, and self-regulation.

THE FOURTH STAGE OF HEALING:
THE GIFT OF SERVICE

This stage of healing (see chapter 8, step 9) is not about healing the already healed hero or heroine of our story. It is about his or her duty to serve the unhealed world and its people. Complete healing is not possible for any of us until all of us, including our planet, are healed. Perhaps the most significant awareness that will emerge from PNI is the recognition that the mind has the capacity not only to regulate our own physiology, but also, because of the effect of one person's mind on another and the even greater effect of the attitudes and beliefs of powerful leaders on the minds of many, it is possible for one person to "control" the physiology and actions of many others. In this sense, the health of all of us and the health of our planet are inextricably con-nected. Those who journey through the healing process must rejoin day-to-day life renewed and affirmed as the authentic healers we so desperately crave.

It is not possible to facilitate the healing of another individual beyond the level of one's own healing. The healer who has journeyed through his or her own healing process understands in the only way possible, through direct experience, the essential nature of healing. Conventional and alternative medicine, primitive and folk healing practices, religious and mystery healings are all connected and con-tained within the panoramic process of healing. Each is a manifestation of one or more aspects of the four stages of healing described above. The healer neither promotes nor assails any healing process that contributes to the movement from external to internal, personal to universal, form to formless, and back again.

It is never easy for an individual who possesses deeper knowledge than those around him or her to function within society. His or her wisdom is intangible, and his or her gifts are noticeable only to those who seek them. To others, they are hidden. Frequently scorned and infrequently honored, such a person models wisdom and harmony and is one to seek out for counsel. His or her task is to maintain centeredness and balance in an uncentered and imbalanced world. He or she must bridge both worlds—inner and outer, form and formless.

At one time or another, we have each met individuals who have facilitated our ability to feel ourselves, for however briefly, as fully alive, vibrant, healthy, and whole. Unfortunately we too often mistake the messenger for the message and assume that the individual alone has opened our hearts and permitted us to catch a glimpse of wholeness and health. Rather than attach ourselves to the healing process that will allow us to live this experience at all times, we attach ourselves to the messenger believing him/her to be the source of our brief dance with aliveness, thus assuring that the joy of wholeness will quickly be replaced by the pain of loss. The source, briefly glanced, can permanently be uncovered only through engaging the four stages of healing. Only then will we discover what is possible for every one of us.

In Nietzsche's words what is possible is for "man to overcome man." Who is this person to be overcome? He or she is the person who lives automatically and mechanically, suffering from distress and dis-ease. The person whose attitudes and ideas, choices and actions are predetermined by the conditioning and programming of his or her mind. It is the person who is deluded into believing that he or she is free when he or she is in fact chained to his mind and body, that he or she loves when he or she is desperately attempting to meet his or her unmet childhood needs, that he or she is joyous when he or she is experiencing momentary pleasures that numb his or her underlying suffering, that he or she can achieve health by treating his or her mind and body as if they were machines in need of repair, and finally that he or she is whole and completed when the sad truth is that he or she is only a fragment of what is possible. This is the person that must be overcome. Not by health professionals, religious men, gurus or others but by him- or herself.

And who exactly is this person who is to "overcome man"? The yogis say he or she is the *I am*, the deeper more essential self freed from the compelling imperatives of the programmed mind we call our personality. The Buddhists call him or her the *no-self*, that which remains when we leave our mind-talk behind and directly experience and bring to our daily lives the noncognitive mindful state of meditation. Buber calls him the *thou*. Maslow refers to him as *self-actualized*. I have spoken of him as the *healed man*. Throughout history all wise men have spoke of this *man*, and there is a place in each of us that knows precisely of what I am speaking. We have all had brief glimpses, moments of astounding clarity, peacefulness, and wholeness, when we have transcended the desires, aversions, worries, fears, and day-to-day details of life to experience a larger more universal self that is neither contaminated nor limited by our conditioned personalities. In these moments we overcome that aspect of humans that directly ascends from the animal kingdom and touch into those uniquely human qualities that stand in relationship to the divine.

This process of overcoming is the process of healing. To engage and sustain it requires the patience, effort, and persistence of which I have spoken in this book: the development of the capacities of mindfulness and self-regulation. It can be so difficult to accomplish that, at times, it seems impossible, and we choose to fall back into our mechanized lives. It is that fragment of its possibility, however, that is our divine spark. It is our greatness. It defines what it means to be fully human, fully healthy, and fully alive.

Now, unlike any other moment or time in history, we are capable of orchestrating our personal and planetary future, creating it as we wish it to be. The pioneering research in PNI and the research to come will continue to demythologize the ancient mysteries and esoteric knowledge of the mystics, making available to each of us all that we need to know to live lives that are worthy of the extraordinary gifts bestowed upon us: the capacity for freedom, joy, truth, and love. These gifts, however, *must* be earned. To claim them we are required to listen carefully, awaken from deep sleep, make the effort and do the work. There is so much more than we have imagined, so much more possible for ourselves, our children, and the planet. There never was and never will be a better time than now.

NOTES

Chapter 1

1. Kirkpatrick, Richard A. "Witchcraft and Lupus Erythematosus." *JAMA*, vol. 245, no. 19, May 1981.

Chapter 2

1. Ader, Robert and Cohen, Nicholas. "Behaviorally Conditioned Immnunosuppression." *Psychosomatic Medical*, vol. 37, no. 4, 1975.
2. Klopfer, Bruno. "Psychological Variables in Human Cancer." Presidential address delivered at the annual meeting of the Society for Projective Techniques, August 31, 1957, New York.
3. Pert, Candace. "The Wisdom of the Receptors: Neuropeptides, the Emotions, and Bodymind." *Advances, Institute for the Advancement of Health*, vol. 3, no. 3, Summer 1986.
4. *Ibid.*
5. Kiecolt-Glaser, Janice, et. al. "Psychological Modifiers of Immunocompetence in Medical Students." *Psychosomatic Medicine*, vol. 46, no. 1, Jan./Feb. 1984.
6. Schnall, Peter L. "The Relationship between 'Job Strain' in Workplace Diastolic Blood Pressure and Left Ventricular Mass Index." *JAMA*, vol. 263, p. 1929, April 1990.

7. Schleiffer, S. J. and Keller, S. E., et. al. "Suppression of Lymphocyte Stimulation During Bereavement." *JAMA*, vol. 250, p. 374, 1983.
8. Kiecolt-Glaser, Janice. "Marital Quality, Marital Disruption, and Immune Function." *Psychosomatic Medicine*, vol. 49, no. 1, Jan./Feb. 1987.
9. Kiecolt-Glaser, Janice and Glaser, Ronald. "Psychological Influences on Immunity." *American Psychologist*, Nov. 1988.

Chapter 4

1. Schultz, Johannes H. "The Clinical Importance of 'Inward Seeing' in Autogenic Training." *British Journal of Medical Hypnotism*, 11-26-28, 1960.
2. Patel, Chandra, et. al. *British Medical Journal*, vol. 200, no. 13, April 1985.
3. Ornish, Dean, et. al. "The Lifestyle Heart Trial." *Lancet*, 336: 129-33, 1990.
4. Blair, Steven, et al. "Physical Fitness and Incidence of Hypertension in Healthy Nonretensive Men and Women." *JAMA*, vol. 252, no. 4, July 1984.

Chapter 5

1. Holmes, Thomas H. and Rahe, Richard H. "The Social Readjustment Rating Scale." *Journal of Psychosomatic Research*, 11: 213–218, 1967.
2. Kobasa, Suzanne. *Journal of Personality and Social Psychology*, vol. 37, pp. 1–10, June 1979.
3. Seyle, Hans. *The Stress of Life* (New York: McGraw Hill, 1978).

Chapter 6

1. Leaf, Alexander and Ryan, Thomas J. "Prevention of Coronary Artery Disease." *New England Journal of Medicine*, vol. 323, pp. 1416–18, Nov. 1990.

Chapter 7

1. Maier, Steven F. and Laudenslager, Mark L. "Inescapable Shock Controllability and Mitogen Stimulated Lymphocyte Proliferation." *Brain, Behavior and Immunity*, vol. 2, no. 2, June 1988.

Chapter 9

1. Cummings, N., et al. "The 20 Year Kaiser Permanent Experience with Psychotherapy and Medical Utilization." *Health Policy Quarterly*, vol. 1, no. 2, 1981.
2. Elite, A. E. "Stress Management Program: RFP Background Paper." Internal paper, California Department of Mental Health, July 1986.
3. Raymond, C. A. "Mental Stress: Occupational Injury of the 80s That Even Pilots Can't Rise Above." *JAMA*, 259: 3097–8, 1988.
4. Fielding, Jonathan. "Worksite Health Promotion and Stress Management." *Advances*, vol. 6, no. 1, pp. 36–40, Spring 1989.

BIBLIOGRAPHY

Recommending books, periodicals, or organizations has never been easy for me. My approach is only to recommend what I have personally experienced and know to be of value. This means that the listings in this appendix are *not* complete. There are many other resources that are of value. This is, however, a good place to begin.

Chapter 1: THE LIMITS OF MODERN MEDICINE: FRONTIERS OF HEALING

Aesclepius. *A Collection and Interpretation of the Testimonies*, Volume I and II. Edelstein E. and L. Arno Press, New York, 1975.

> These volumes are the definitive work on the Aesclepian healing temples. The authors provide us with a full account of the development, practices, and significance of temple medicine. This information is supported by transcriptions of the many testimonials inscribed in stone and left at the temples and the written commentaries of writers and important figures of the time.

Star, P. *The Social Transformation of American Medicine*. Basic Books, New York, 1982.

> This scholarly book traces the development of American medicine, as a profession and industry, from the mid-eighteenth century to the present

date. It discusses the successes, failures, and future directions of our health-care system. If you have a special interest in a more detailed understanding of these issues, this book can serve as a good resource.

Ardell, D. *High Level Wellness*. Ten Speed Press, Berkeley, 1986.

In this early, and more recently revised discussion of "wellness," the author provides us with a concise, and well-presented introduction to the concepts and practices of wellness.

Travis, J. and Ryan, R. *The Wellness Workbook*. Ten Speed Press, Berkeley, 1988.

In this book, the founder of the wellness movement, Dr. Travis, and his associate, present their views on the important issues and aspects of well-ness. Topics include among others: breathing, sensing, finding meaning, playing, feeling, and working.

Smuts, J. *Holism and Evolution*. Greenwood Press Publishers, Westport, 1926, 1973.

This scholarly work is the first, and still the most definitive, exploration and discussion of the concept of holism.

Chapter 2: PSYCHONEUROIMMUNOLOGY: RECONNECTING MIND AND BODY

Locke, S., M.D. and Colligan, D. *The Healer Within*. E. P. Dutton, New York, 1986.

This easy-to-read book, written by a prominent researcher in the field of PNI, demystifies the science of PNI, explores its implications for contempo-rary medicine, and provides the reader with helpful advice on mind-body healing.

Chapter 3: MINDFULNESS

Goldstein, J. *The Experience of Insight*. Shambala, Boulder, 1987.

This is an important book. It is a detailed introduction to the practice of mindfulness. It is clear, concise, and greatly expands upon the information in this chapter.

Goldstein, J. and Kornfield, J. *Seeking the Heart of Wisdom*. Shambala, Boston and London, 1987.

This is a companion book to *The Experience of Insight*. Well written and highly recommended, it expands upon the previously presented concepts, drawing the reader into an increasingly deeper understanding of mindfulness.

Kornfield, J. and Breiter, P. *A Still Forest Pool, The Insight Meditation of Achaan Chah*. The Theosophical Publishing House, Wheaton, 1985.

This wonderful, sweet book introduces the reader to the wisdom of mindfulness as expressed by a skilled teacher and wise man. The writing is clear, the little parables wonderful, and, in time, you begin to assimilate the feeling and teachings of the monastic life, much of which is applicable to modern-day living.

Chapter 4: SELF-REGULATION

Green, E. and A. *Beyond Biofeedback*. Delta, New York, 1977.

This wonderful, readable, and wise book, written by the pioneers of biofeedback and self-regulation, is filled with research data, personal experiences, and clinical observations. The authors review topics such as homeostasis, self-regulation, biofeedback training, the role of biofeedback in the treatment of specific disorders, body consciousness, mind training, and volition.

Chapter 5: ACHIEVING GENERAL RELAXATION

This information is contained in books already listed.

Chapter 6: REGULATING THE BODY

Anderson, B. *Stretching*. Shelter Publications, Bolinas, 1980.

This is an excellent guide to stretching. It begins with a simple ten-minute daily stretch routine, and expands to provide a more focused routine for different muscle groups. Like aerobic conditioning, the correct approach to stretching is not necessarily what you learn from following others. It is well worth the time to learn to do it right.

Cooper, K. *The Aerobics Way*. Bantam, New York, 1977.

Very few individuals who "work out" know much about the practical aspects of aerobic conditioning. The information in this book teaches you how to use your workout most effectively by training yourself effectively, efficiently, and safely.

Chapter 7: REGULATING THE MIND

Refer to the readings recommended for chapter 4.

Swami Hariharananda Aranya. *The Yoga Philosophy of Patanjali*. State University of New York Press, Albany, 1983.

> This book is not for everyone. It requires much time with each word, sentence, and paragraph, as well as considerable patience with a new vocabulary. The reward is equal to the task. This book commonly referred to as the *Yoga Sutras*, is a complete science of the mind. It is a detailed description of how the mind works and how to work with it.

Starr, A. *Solitude, A Return to Self*. Free Press, New York, 1988.

> Although a bit erudite, this book examines an important, and infrequently discussed, issue. Contrary to the perspectives of western society, which often measures well-being by the capacity to succeed in relationships, Storr makes the case that true health and happiness results from the capacity to live at peace with oneself. He explores the relationship of solitude to creativity, self-growth, healing, and the religious experience.

Johnson, R. *We*. Harper and Row, Cambridge, 1983.

> This marvelous short book explores the western notion of romance. It examines the relationship of romance to the practical and spiritual aspects of life. Through the classical story of Tristan and Isolde, he suggests answers to our recurring questions about the role of intimate relationships in our lives.

Fromm, E. *The Art of Loving*. Harper and Row, New York, 1956.

> In this classic work, the author, in a concise, simple, and wise manner, discusses the nature of love and provides a practical set of guidelines that may assist individuals in creating healthy loving relationships.

Chapter 8: WORKING THE PROGRAM

This information is contained in books already listed.

Chapter 9: NAVIGATING THE HEALTH-CARE SYSTEM

Needleman, J. *The Way of the Physician*. Harper and Row, San Francisco, 1985.

The author examines the predicaments, ideals, and challenges of modern medicine and the physicians who practice it. He looks towards the future and explores how we can recapture the ideals and humanism of medicine. It is wonderful reading filled with personal recollections, up-to-date knowledge, and the wisdom of this philosopher.

Chapter 10: THE FOUR STAGES OF HEALING

Campbell, Joseph, *The Hero with a Thousand Faces*, Princeton University Press, Princeton, 1949.

In this seminal work, Campbell synthesizes his extraordinary knowledge of mythology, religion, and literature into a model of human growth and development. This book is wise and inspiring.

Suggested Reading

Berry, T. *The Dream of the Earth.* Sierra Club Books, San Francisco, 1988.

This wonderful and scholarly book makes a compelling case for the earth. Many important facts and issues are presented. The author, urging us to consider ourselves as a vanguard of the next era, the ecologic era, describes a step-by-step approach to global healing. This is an important book to read.

Daumal, R. *Mount Analogue.* Shambala, Boston, 1986.

One of my favorites. Mountains are metaphors for the connection between the earth and the heavens. In this marvelous story, Daumal teaches us about the journey to wholeness: the ascent, the plateaus, the obstacles, the challenges, and the rewards. It is short, concise, and beautifully written.

Miller, A. *Death of a Salesman.* Penguin Books, New York, 1976.

This work is the great tragic drama of the modern era. Miller offers us the sad story of Willy Loman's life, a life lived on "automatic pilot." He also offers us the hope in Willy's son, Biff.

Eliot, T. S. *Selected Poems.* Harcourt, Brace, Jovanovich, New York, 1934.

This selection contains "The Wasteland" and "The Hollow Men," two of Eliot's finest poems, which express the cost to society when it substitutes materialism and instant gratification for sensitivity, mindfulness, and spirituality.

Krishnamurti, J. *Freedom From the Known*. Harper and Row, New York, 1969.

One reads Krishnamurti to experience his extraordinary analysis of the problems of modern times and his precise, brilliant, and mindful mind. In this book, he explores the issue of personal freedom, which he believes develops as we shift from a conditioned mind, that lives from the past to a creative mind that lives in the here and now. It is an excellent complement to the other readings on insight and mindfulness.

Thoreau, H. D. *Walden*. Doubleday, New York, 1954.

Whitman, W. *Leaves of Grass*. Doubleday, New York, 1960.

In these American classics, Thoreau and Whitman demonstrate an extraordinary capacity for mindfulness. Whitman's observations of the experiences of daily life, and Thoreau's observations about solitude and nature are inspiring examples of how to live a mindful life.

PERIODICALS

Advances, Fetzer Institute 9292 West KL Avenue, Kalamazoo, MI 49009.

This quarterly publication and occasional supplemental mailings has as their goal, "the expansion and communication of knowledge about the integration of mind and body in health and disease." The articles, book reviews, and calendar of events are good sources of information for individuals who wish a continuous update on current issues in mind-body healing.

Nutrition Action, Center for Science in the Public Interest, 1501 16th Street, NW, Washington, DC 20077.

This is the best up-to-date, reliable, well-presented source of nutrition information I have found. The monthly magazine and the variety of valuable posters and booklets provide the subscriber with a comprehensive set of resources.

Parabola, The Society of Myth and Tradition, 656 Broadway, New York, NY 10012.

This beautiful, informative, and highly inspirational magazine explores a different topic each quarter. Contributing writers offer their comments on topics such as wholeness, the hero, disciples and discipline, addiction, forgiveness, and many others.

University of California, Berkeley Wellness Letter, P.O. Box 420148, Palm Coast, FL 32142.

This monthly newsletter offers its readers a variety of articles on nutrition, fitness, and stress management. Its focus is on prevention.

RESOURCES

Insight Meditation Society, Pleasant Street, Barre, MA 01001.
Insight Meditation West, P.O. Box 909, Woodacre, CA 94973.

Both of these organizations offer three-, ten-, thirty-, and ninety-day intensive mindfulness meditation retreats. These retreats are an opportunity for intensive study under the guidance of skilled teachers. They are highly recommended for both beginners and advanced students.

Commonweal, P.O. Box 316, Bolinas, CA 94924.

This is an education and training center that assists individuals with cancer to explore complementary forms of healing that will enable the individual to work with cancer more effectively to maximize self-healing and "expand" life. This program is highly recommended.

The Krishnamurti Foundation, P.O. Box 1560, Ojai, California 94924

This organization continues the work of Krishnamurti (see bibliography). They offer a variety of programs, retreats, and educational materials related to mindfulness and self-healing.

Esalen Institute, Big Sur, CA 93920.
The Omega Institute, Lake Drive R.D. 2, Box 377, Rhinebeck, NY.

The Kripalu Center, P.O. Box 793, Lenox, MA 01240.
The New York Open Center, 83 Spring Street, New York, NY 10012.
Interface, 552 Main Street, Watertown, MA 02172.

Each of these centers provides a variety of programs dealing with issues such as meditation, health and healing, movement, personal development, Yoga, and environment and global issues.

INDEX

A

Abundance, 145–148
  observing deprivation and
    abundance; exercise, 148–
    149
Ader, Robert, 16
Aerobic conditioning, 94, 101
  and the heart, 98
Aeschylus, 4
Aesclepias, 3, 5
Aging process, 66
AIDS, 110
Air pollution, 95
Air, Water, and Places, 13
Alcoholics Anonymous (AA), 183
  holistic approach of, 6
"Allegory of the Cave," 121
Aloneness, 140
Alzheimer's disease, 67
American Psychologist, emotional stress
  and infection, 23
Anger, 122–123
  repressed; physiological effect on
    body, 25

Antibody mediated immunity, 109
Arteries, 95–96
Arthritis, 111
The Art of Loving, 133
Asanas, 70
Atherosclerosis, 96, 97
  and heart disease, 86, 97–98
  plaques, 101
Attention, 34–35
  exercise, 45–47
Attitude, 37–38
Autoimmune diseases, 111
Autonomic nervous system (ANS),
  17–18, 96–97

B

Balance, 119
  maintenance of in mind-body
    healing program, 164
B cells, 108, 109f
Behavioral conditioning, 16
Benson, Herbert, 59
Beta-endorphin, 19
The Bhagavad Gita excerpt, 55

Biofeedback, 23, 29, 58–59, 63, 101
The Birth of Venus, 134–135
Blair, Steven, 65
Body
  communication systems of, 17–24,
    18f
  regulation of. *See* Regulating the
    body
  self-regulation of, 65–66
Bortz, Walter M., 65–66
Botticelli, 134–135
Bowels, self-regulation of, 107–108
Bradshaw, John, 75
Breathing, 50–51
  complete (diaphragmatic), 78f, 79,
    95
  controlled; exercise, 77–81, 92–
    95
  inadequate, 89–90
  timed, 79
  see also Respiratory system
British Medical Journal, paper on
    general relaxation, 64
Buber, Martin, 196
Buddhists, 195

C

California Workman's Compensation
    Institute, stress-related claims,
    178
Campbell, Joseph, 188
Cancer, 65
  colonic, 104
  innovative treatment programs,
    115–116
  mind-body healing, 16–17
  in patients with loss and loneliness,
    111
  research and therapy, 110–111
Cannon, Walter B., 57–58
Carbon dioxide, 88, 89
Cardiac arrhythmias, 23
Cardiovascular system
  conditioning, 98
  disease of, 65

  mindfulness, increased; exercise,
    99–102
Central nervous system (CNS), 17,
    18
Childhood woundings, 71, 123, 148
Cholesterol, 98
Chronic pain syndromes, 72
Circulatory system, 95–102
  the broken heart, 96–99
  cardiovascular system, 98–102
  diet, 101
  self-regulation of, 58, 97, 101
Colon cancer, 104
Community, 169
  healing, 182–183
Companionship, importance of, 22–
    23
Concentration, 35, 192
  exercise, 47–49
  mindful, 83
Conscious living, 60–61, 168
  balance, 119
  contentment, 119–120
  harmlessness, 120
  honesty, 120
  as part of mind-body healing
    program, 161–162
  simplicity, 120
  solitude, 120–121
Contentment, 119–120
Corporations
  styles of, 179
  wellness, interest in, 12
  worksite, 178–181
Creativity and imagery, 83
Crohn's disease, 104
Cytoxan, 16

D

Daily living, 60–61
  environment; modification of, 183–
    184
  keeping a journal, 168
Dairy products, 94
Demoralization, 72

Deprivation, 118, 144–151
  abundance, 145–148
  observing deprivation and
      abundance; exercise, 148–149
  remembering; exercise, 149–151
Diet and nutrition, 83–84
  for the bowels, 107–108
  and the circulatory system, 101
  and the gastrointestinal system,
      104
  and the immune system, 116
Disease, 58
  modern medicine's focus on, 1–2
  predisposing factors, 155–156
  the role of stress in, 11, 70
Diverticulosis, 104–105
  Dunn, Halbert, 12
Dyslexia, 67

E

Eating; mindfulness exercise, 54–56
Eliot, T. S., 36
Emotions, 20–21
  and physiology, 21
Environment
  air pollution, 95
  healing, 183–184
  inner and outer, 57
  and well-being, 156
Euripides, 4
Exercises
  for the cardiovascular system;
      increased mindfulness, 99–
      102
  for the gastrointestinal system,
      106–108
  for general relaxation, 74–84
      controlled breathing, 77–81
      guided imagery, 82–83
      tense-relax, 75–77
  for learning mindfulness, 40–56
      attention, 45–47
      concentration, 47–49
      in daily living, 54–56
      eating, 54–56

  for individuals with a restless
      mind, 54–55
      meditation, 49–50
      mindfulness, 45–53
      mind-talk, 41–45
      training yourself, 51–53
  for mindful relationships, 141–
      144
  for remembering, 149–151
  for the respiratory system
      controlled breathing, 92–95
      mindfulness, 90–92
      powerlessness, 128–131, 131–
      133
  to enhance awareness of the
      immune system, 112–114
  to observe deprivation and
      abundance, 148–149

F

Factual information, 32–33
The Family, 75
Feelings, 43
Fight-or-flight response, 72–73
The Four Quartets excerpt, 36
Fromm, Erich, 133

G

Gastrointestinal system, 102–108
  diet, 104
  exercise for, 106–108
  upset stomach, 103–106
Genetic predisposition, 67–68, 104,
      111
  and well-being, 156
Glaser, Ronald, 23
Greece, ancient
  Aesclepian healing temples, *xiv*
  holistic view, 5–6
  tragedies, 4–5
  see also Temple healing
Green, Elmer and Alyce, 58–59
Guided imagery and the immune
      system, 115–116

H

Habits, 60
Hardiness, 70
Harmlessness, 120
Hashimoto's thyroid disease, 111
Healed man, 196
Healers and healing
  attitudinal healing, 116
  beginning of, 156
  communities, 182–183
  components of, 30f
    see also Mindfulness; Self-
      regulation
  defined, 10
  distress, directed at sources of, 11
  the individual's role, 10
  mind-body healing program. *See*
      Mind-body healing program
  in mindfulness, 38
  nature of, *xiv*
  setting of, 10
  stages of, 189–196
    see also Stages of healing
  treatment versus, 10–11
  see also Temple healing
Health-care system
  healing communities, 182–183
  healing environments, 183–184
  mind-body healing practiced within
      constraints of, 174
  navigation of, 171–188
  practitioner and client, 172–175
Health care systems, 185–186
  aims beyond accommodation, 186–
    187
  the healing self, 185–186
  mind-body healing of tomorrow,
      center for, 187–188
Health insurance carriers, 174, 175–
    177
  considerations when choosing a
      plan, 177
  getting the most from,
      recommendations for, 177–
      178

mental health benefits, 178
  options, 176
Health Maintenance Organization
    (HMO)
  fixed panel versus open panel,
      176
  physician's role in, *xiii–xiv*
  providers of, 176–177
Heart, diseases of, 96–97
Heart attack, 96, 97
Heart disease, 62–63
  atherosclerotic, 86
  and life-style interventions, 86
  and relaxation practices, 64, 65
Herpes virus, 23
High Level Wellness, 12
Hippocrates, 13
Holism and Evolution, 13
Holistic healing, 13–14
  in ancient Greece, 5–6
  "holism" defined, 13
Holmes, Thomas H., 70
Homecoming, 75
Homeostasis, 57–58
  and the immune system, 111
  nasal heat exchange system, 87
Honesty, 120
Hormonal system, 19–20
Hospitals
  as healing environments, 183
  wellness, interest in, 12
Humidification, 94
Huntington's Chorea, 67
Huxley, Aldous, 56
Hypertension, 96–97, 98, 178
  white coat hypertension, 97

I

I am, 195
Imagery, 44
  and creativity, 83
  guided; exercise for, 82–83
  mental, 23, 44
  visual, 8
Immune cells, 19

Immune function, and stress, 22
Immune system, 108–117
  antibody mediated immunity,
    109
  attitudinal healing, 116
  B cells, 108, 109f
  disordered immunity, 110–112
  and exercise, 115
  exercises to enhance awareness of,
    112–114
  and guided imagery, 115–116
  and homeostasis, 111
  natural killer cells, 108, 109f
  and nutrition, 116
  and powerlessness, 125
  and relaxation, 114–115
  self-regulation of, 114–117
  and sleep deprivation, 117
  and social support, 117
  and stress, 73
  T cells, 108, 109f
Infection and stress, 23–24
Irritable bowel syndrome, 104–105
Island excerpt, 56

J

Job search; questions to ask before
    accepting a new position,
    180
Job strain, 64, 97
  JAMA article on physiologic effects
    of, 22
  treatment techniques, 181
John's healing of ulcerative colitis, 7–
    9, 24–26
  mind-body disorder of, 27f
  physician/patient roles in healing
    process, 28
  recent changes in his life, 28–29
  recommendations for, 28
Journal of the American Medical
    Association (JAMA)
  job strain, physiologic effects, 22
  life-style intervention and heart
    disease, 86

lupus, report of mind-body healing
    of, 6

K

Kaiser Permanente, 176
Kaposi's sarcoma, 110
Kiecolt-Glaser, Janice K., 22, 23
Klopfer, Bruno, 16
Kobassa, Suzanne, 70
Krebiozen, 16–17

L

Lancet, life-style intervention and
    heart disease, 86
Large intestine, 103
Laudenslager, Mark, 125
Leaf, Alexander, 86–87
Learning, state-dependent, 25
Life-style interventions, 86
Living. See Conscious living; Daily
    living
Loneliness and loss, 22–23, 118,
    133–144
  and cancer, 111
  love, a different kind of, 136–137
  mindful relationships; exercise,
    141–144
  relationship, skills of, 137–141
Love, 133, 135, 140
  a different kind of, 136–137
  self-love, 134–135, 137–138
Lupus
  JAMA report of mind-body healing
    of, 6–7
  systemic, 111

M

Maier, Steven, 125
Marbach, Joseph, 72
Marital quality, 23
Mary's powerlessness, healing of, 126–
    128
Maslow, 196

Medicine
  focus on disease, 1–2
  illness and exam, modern routine
    of, 2–3
  limits of modern medicine, 1–14
  modern practice of, *xiii–xiv*, 1–14,
    174, 190
  as a part of healing, *xv*
  technology, role of, 7, 9
  see also Patient/physician
    relationship
Meditation, 35–36, 165
  exercise, 49–50
  transcendental, 59–60
Memory, 32
  remembering; exercise, 149–151
Mental imagery
  effect on heart rhythm, 23
  images, 44
Mental states, effect on neuropeptides,
    20f, 20–21
The mind
  activities of. *See* Mind-talk;
    Mindfulness
  as part of the human organism, 71–
    72
  regulation of. *See* Regulating the
    mind
  self-regulation of, 66–67
  workings of, 36f, 71–73
Mind-body healing
  language difficulties, 26, 28–29
  physical aspects of disease, view of,
    24
  see also Psychoneuroimmunology
Mind-body healing program, 153–170
  the first year, 165–166
  process of, 154f, 156
  steps in the program, 158–165
    basic mindfulness and self-
      regulation, 160–161
    breakthrough to wholeness, 164–
      165
    conscious living, 161–162
    establishing a healing
      environment, 160

knowing treatment from healing,
    159
  maintaining balance, 164
  mastering mindfulness, 162–163
  mastering self-regulation, 163
  the search for improvement, 159
  serving others, 165
Mindfulness, *xvi*, 30f, 30–56, 31f
  alternatives to, 56
  aspects of, 31, 34–36
  basic understanding of as part of
    healing program, 160–161
  development of, 37
  difficulties in maintaining, 157
  exercises, 45–53
  goals of, 37
  healing stress by. *See* Exercises, for
    general relaxation
  and inner abundance, 147
  mastering technique in healing
    program, 162–163
  mind, workings of, 31–37
  self-regulation compared to, 63,
    121–124
  and stress, 62
  training, 37–40
    see also Attitude; Exercises for
      learning mindfulness;
      Patience; Solitude
Mind-talk, 31f, 31–32
  aspects of, 31
  defined, 71
  development of, 32f
  exercise, 41–45
  stored information, reliance on, 33
  unhealthy, 71
Mucus production, 94
  excessive, 89

N

National Council on Compensation
    Insurance, stress-related
    claims, 179
National Institutes of Health (NIH),
    PNI Unit, 15

Natural killer cells, 108, 109f, 109–
        110
Neuropeptides, 17, 113–114
    beta-endorphin, 19
    discovery of, 18–21
    implications of discovery of, 21
    mental state, effect on, 20f, 20–21
    receptors in the gastrointestinal
        system, 104
    system, 19f
    transmitters, 73
New England Journal of Medicine, life-
        style intervention and heart
        disease, 86–87
No-self, 195–196
Nutrition. See Diet and nutrition

O

Obsession, 71
O'Connor, Gerald T., 98
Ode: Intimations of Immortality excerpt
        (Wordsworth), 146
Opiates, brain cell receptors of, 18–
        19
Ornish, Dean, 65, 86
Osler, Wiliam, 13
Oxygen, 88

P

Papyrus Didotrana, 4
Past experience, importance of, 33
    see also Mind-talk
Patel, Chandra, 64
Patience, 39–40
Patient
    as a consumer of medical care, 2–3
    "worried well," 3
    see also Patient/physician
        relationship
Patient/physician relationship, xv
    appointment and physical exam,
        2–3
    commitment of healer, 173
    in the health-care system, 172–175

health professional's basic
        philosophy, 172
    in John's healing process (ulcerative
        colitis), 28
    nature of healer, 173
    training of healer, 173
Phidias, 4
Physical fitness, 65
    aerobic conditioning, 94
    and the immune system, 115
    physiological effects of exercise, 65–
        66
Physiology and emotion, 21
Plato, 121
Powerlessness, 118, 124–133
    grieving our losses; exercise, 131–
        133
    and the immune system, 125
    inner power; exercise, 128–131
    inner power, 126–128
Pranayama, 70
Praxiteles, 4
Preferred provider organization (PPO),
        177
Psychologic information, 32, 33
Psychoneuroimmunology (PNI), xv–
        xvi, 15–29
    development of, 16–17
    stress and the immune system, 73
    see also Mind-body healing

R

Rahe, Richard H., 70
Regulating the body, 85–117
    circulatory system, 95–102
    gastrointestinal system, 102–108
    the immune system, 108–117
    the respiratory system, 87–95
Regulating the mind, 118–152
    conscious living, 119–121
    deprivation, 144–151
    loneliness, 133–144
    mindfulness as self-regulation, 121–
        124
    powerlessness, 124–133

Relationships, 136–137, 169
  aloneness, 140–141
  defined, 140–141
  difference is not rejection, 139
  giving, 138
  intimate, 144
  mindful; exercise, 141–144
  need to change in, 140
  self-love, 137–138
  separateness is not withdrawal,
      139–140
  skills of, 137–141
Relaxation, 69–84
  and heart disease, 64, 65
  and the immune system, 114–
      115
  and self-regulation, 64–65
  techniques, 8, 24–25
  see also Exercises for general
      relaxation
Research, current, 22–24
Respiratory system, 87–95
  controlled breathing exercise, 92–
      95
  daily regulation of, practices to
      assist in, 94–95
  inhalation and exhalation, 88–89
  mechanics of, 87–89
  mindfulness of; exercise, 90–92
  respiratory distress, 89–90
  see also Breathing; Exercises, for
      the respiratory system

S

Schizophrenia, 67
Schleiffer, Steven, 22–23
Schnall, Peter L., 22, 97
Schultz, Johannes H., 58
Self-healing, 29, 185–186
  fifty ways to begin, 166–169
Self-knowledge, xiv–xv
Self-love, 134–135, 137–138
Self-regulation, xvi, 30f, 57–68
  application of, 63–67
  appropriateness, 62

aspects of, 62–63
basic understanding of, as part of
    healing program, 160–161
and biofeedback, 63
of the body, 65–66
capacity for, 163
of the circulatory system, 58, 97,
    101
components of, 60–61
conscious living, 60–61
daily practices, 60–61
and general relaxation, 64–65
healing stress by. See Exercises for
    general relaxation
of heart disease, 62–63
human capacity for, 58
of the immune system, 114–117
limits of, 67–68
mastering technique in healing
    program, 162–163
measurability, 62, 63
of the mind, 66–67
mindfulness compared to, 63, 121–
    124
summarized, 67f
system diagram, 59f
through biofeedback, 58–59
timeliness, 62
see also Mindfulness
Selye, Hans, 72–73
Sensations, 43
Sensory system, 31–32
Service to others, 165, 194–196
Sex, 137
Sickle-cell anemia, 67, 157
Silence, 191
Simplicity, 120
Sleep deprivation, 117
Small intestine, 103
Smoking, 89, 98
Smuts, Jan, 13
Social support, 117
Solitude, 38–39, 120–121, 191
Sophocles, 4
Space, external and internal, 80
Spastic colitis, 104–105

Stages of healing, 189–196
  healing at the source, 191–192
  service to others, 194–196
  symptoms, working with, 190–191
  wisdom, wholeness, and full health,
    192–194
Steroids, 73
Steve's mild depression, healing of,
  124–126
Stomach, upset, 103–106
Stress
  at the worksite, 179, 181
  components of, 26, 28
  and disease, 11, 70
  fight-or-flight response, 72–73
  healing by mindfulness and self-
    regulation, 74–84
    see also Exercises, for general
    relaxation
  historic methods of handling, 69
  and the immune system, 22, 73
  and infection, 23–24
  insurance claims for; statistics, 178,
    179
  job-related. See Job strain
  and mindfulness, 62
  the mind's role in, 71
  options in coping with, 62
Stressors, 72
Symptoms
  complexes, 3
  physical, 2
  working with, 190–191

T

T cells, 108, 109f, 109
Temperomandibular joint (TMJ) pain,
  72
Temple healing, 3–6
  decision to journey to temple, 4
  elements in modern society, 6–9
  fundamental approach, 5–6
  Greek tragedies, 4–5
  purification process, 4–5

  return to health, 5
  testimonials etched in stone, 4
Thou, 196
Thoughts, 42
Tintern Abbey excerpt, 36
Transcendental Meditation (TM), 59–
  60
Travis, John, 12, 13
Treatment
  defined, 10
  healing versus, 10–11
  setting of, 10
  technology of, 9

U

Ulcerative colitis, 104
  John's healing of, 7–9, 24–26, 27–
    29

V

Vasculitis, 111
Veins, 96
Veterans Administration hospital,
    student diagnosis at, 1–2
Visual imagery, 8

W

Wellness, 12–13
  corporate interest in, 12
  modern application of, 13–14
Witch doctor, 6
Wordsworth, William, 36, 146
Worksite, 178–181
  stress, causes of and treatment
    techniques, 179, 181
"Worried well" patients, 3

Y

Yoga, 69–70
Yogis, 21, 29, 195
  on happiness, 120

ABOUT THE AUTHOR

Elliott S. Dacher, M.D., currently practices medicine in Reston, Virginia. His practice integrates the traditional elements of an internal medicine practice, diagnosis and treatment, and the innovative components of a self-healing program, mindfulness, and self-regulation.

Dr. Dacher has conducted numerous workshops and seminars for professionals as well as laypeople in the health-care field on the topics of wellness, psychoneuroimmunology, and self-healing. He has consulted and written on these topics and has appeared on numerous radio talk shows.

Dr. Dacher was graduated from the medical school of the State University of New York at Buffalo in 1970. He completed his training in internal medicine in 1975 on the Harvard Medical Service at the Peter Bent Brigham Hospital. He is a certified Diplomate of the American Board of Internal Medicine.

Dr. Dacher currently resides in Reston, Virginia. He has two daughters ages fifteen and twenty. He is currently working on a future book and plans to continue studying, practicing, and teaching on issues related to self-healing.

Q. 2 — 2 way process —

Are the neuropeptides produced in brain same
   as those produced in humoral & immune cells?

Glands are neuropeptides Transmitters?